Sixth Edition

Baby & Me

The Essential Guide to Pregnancy and Newborn Care

Jenny B. Harvey
Deborah D. Stewart

Illustrated by Christine Thomas

Bull Publishing Company
Boulder, Colorado

Text: Copyright © 2025 by Jenny B. Harvey and
    Deborah Davis Stewart
Graphics: Copyright © 2025 by Christine Thomas

Bull Publishing Company
P.O. Box 1377
Boulder, CO 80306
Phone: 800-676-2855
www.bullpub.com

Library of Congress Cataloging-in-Publication Data

Harvey, Jenny B., author.
   Baby and me : the essential guide to pregnancy and newborn
   care / Jenny B. Harvey, Deborah D. Stewart. -- Sixth edition.
      pages cm
   Includes bibliographical references and index.
   ISBN 978-1-945188-59-6 (paperback)

CIP data application in process. Please contact the publisher for more information.

Printed in U.S.A.

29 28 27 26 25   10 9 8 7 6 5 4 3 2 1

Design and production by Dovetail Publishing Services
Cover design by Shannon Bodie, Lightbourne Images

*From Jenny to my sweet Hazel Elizabeth and Violet Louise,
my babies forever and ever. Thank you for sharing so much
of your mama with this book. Love you so!*

*From Deborah to my dear daughter, Cricket, whose birth as a
preemie 55 years ago inspired the first edition of this book, and
my two loving grandsons, as well as to my partner and best
friend, Warren.*

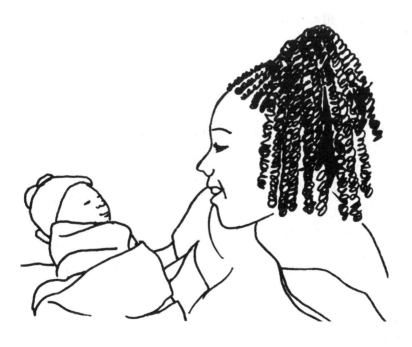

A note to you from Jenny . . .

Welcome to Baby & Me! I'm so glad this book found you. No matter where you are at in your family planning journey, we made this book for you! We've tried to make it easy to read and hope that you'll find what you need to feel good about taking care of your body in the coming years.

Your story is your own. You may be getting ready to have sex for the first time, or just found out that you're pregnant, or maybe you're just days away from meeting your baby. You may be happy and excited, or overwhelmed and not sure what to do. This book is a safe space for you to learn about what's happening and what choices you have to make. I hope that you feel welcome and seen as you read it.

My goal for this book is to offer you unbiased information so that you can make informed choices that feel right to you, even when they are hard. I want you to feel like you understand what's happening, what your providers are talking about, and what your options are. I want to offer support and remind you that you are doing your best and that you are enough.

If you get overwhelmed or aren't sure where to start, go back to the Table of Contents and pick a spot. Or, go to Chapter 17 and browse some of the great websites we have included. Watch videos and make a list of questions you have. Having a healthy family starts with you. I'm rooting for you!

Sending peace, strength, safety, love, patience, and lots of joy!

Jenny Burris Harvey, BA
Seattle, Washington

A note to you from Deborah . . .

Now we have given birth to the sixth edition of Baby & Me, which is very hard for me to believe. My goal since the first version, almost 30 years ago, has always been to help parents have healthy pregnancies and give birth to happy, healthy babies. In some ways this has become easier over the years, with more and more resources for help, such as more midwives and doulas. In other ways, it has become harder, but overall, the more you know the easier your pregnancy will be. Keep your eye on prevention—so many problems are easier to deal with before they get serious.

This book is still devoted to helping you have a healthy baby. The more you can do to prevent problems the better. Here you will find the best basic information about pregnancy, birth, and newborn care, the foundation for a healthy family. But also remember that there is a lot of help available when you need it. Don't be afraid to ask!

Best wishes from my heart. I hope you will be able to enjoy this special time, even if it feels tough sometimes. Remember that you and your body are doing an amazing thing, a true miracle. I'd like to give you a big hug!

Deborah Davis Stewart, BA
Seattle, Washington

Acknowledgments

This sixth edition of Baby & Me has many great updates to important topics, such as family planning, prenatal care, vaccines and germs in pregnancy, creating healthy habits and quitting harmful habits, surgical birth, and infant care.

Special thanks to our wonderful illustrator, Christine Thomas, who was able to create even more incredible images for us on this edition to make sure the information is not only clear to our readers but that it's also welcoming and inclusive.

We are so thankful to each of our reviewers who generously shared their expertise with us for this update. Your insight and feedback is invaluable as we strive to keep this book as up-to-date as possible.

Elias Kass, ND. Naturopathic doctor specializing in the care of babies and children, practicing at Intergalactic Pediatrics, Seattle, Washington

Jeffrey Kerr-Layton, MD

Joy MacTavish, MA, IBCLC, RLC, Certified Holistic Sleep Coach: Owner, Sound Beginnings

Geneva Murphy - Mother, Doula for single Moms, Placenta Encapsulation at Powerful Placenta, Trauma Informed Yoga Teacher , Reiki Practitioner and Self-Care teacher at RainFlower YOGA & Reiki, Neuro Art & Therapeutic Art Facilitator, and a lover of all birth and healing work.

Shamila Panjwani, DO

Virginia Raffaele, PA-C, CD

Sharon Sobers-Outlaw, MSW, MHP, CDP: Clinical social worker, counselor, certified Minority Mental Health Consultant, and certified Behavior Activation Therapist. Advocate for cultural awareness, equity, inclusion, and social justice.

Lastly, continued thanks to the amazing expert reviewers from previous editions whose input remains part of the foundation for this book over the years.

Barbara Decker, Melinda Ferguson, Debra Golden, Betsy Hayford, Benjamin Hoffman, Kim James, Lisa Meuleman, Sharon Muza, Marni B. Port, Linda Ungerleider, Maricela Vega, and Kathy Wilson. And to the many other professionals who shared their insight on breastfeeding, infant care, and safety.

Please note

This book should not be the only guide you use to care for yourself and your unborn child. Your doctor or midwife and other medical professionals are trained to help you take care of yourself. Please consult those who know your special needs.

Contents

Using This Book

If you are pregnant or thinking of getting pregnant, taking care of yourself now is the most important thing you can do to have a healthy, happy baby. This book can help. Take a quick look all the way through it. Then read the chapters again, as your pregnancy moves along.

This book is yours!

Keep it handy and use it often. Highlight or write in it as much as you like. Mark pages you want to go back to. Use the notes pages to keep track of how you feel, questions you have, or things your provider says that you want to remember.

Partners, grandparents, other family members

This book isn't just for moms. Dads, moms, and other partners go through huge changes when getting ready for baby, too. Partners will play a big part in a baby's life, from pregnancy on. So we have created a special place at the end of each chapter with tips just for them. We hope you will share these partner tips, and the rest of the book, with them.

Grandparents and other relatives may play a big role in caring for their grandbabies. Share this book with them. We hope it will help them catch up on the latest best practices in pregnancy, birth, and baby care. Sharing this book may help you talk with them about how they can be a part of this new life.

Traditions in birth and baby care

The advice in this book may be different from what your family or your people have done in the past. Sometimes, people tell you how things should be done simply because that's how they did them. Other times, it is cultural tradition that things are done a certain way. For example, in some cultures, certain foods are not eaten during pregnancy. In others, men do not take part in the birth.

There are many ways to good health, and family values are important. The ideas in this book, which come from the most current science, will give you and your baby a healthy start. If you wish to do something different, talk about it with your doctor, nurse, or midwife. Tell them your reasons or concerns. Listen to what they say. Then decide what you feel is best for you and your baby.

The words we use

All families, parents, and babies are unique. In this book, we have tried to welcome and include all people. We especially want you to know that this book is for you, no matter what age you are, if you have a partner or not, and no matter what gender you or your partner may be.

Medical words

There are many different names for medical people who might care for you. We often will use "healthcare provider" or just "provider" instead of "doctor, midwife, or nurse" in this book.

Medical talk can be confusing. We have tried to use words that are easy to understand. You will find it helpful to learn some medical words, since your provider may use them a lot. When you see a word marked with a star like this*, you can see what it means at the side of that page. Meanings of many words you will need to know are in the glossary at the end of Chapter 17.

Chapter 1

Taking Care of Your Body

Your health is important

Bodies can do amazing things. One of the most important things you can do is learn how to take care of yours. You've already gone through so many changes as you've gotten older, you might already feel like a pro. But, when you start to have sex, there are new ways you need to take care of yourself. And when you may be pregnant, it's even more important to keep yourself safe and healthy.

No matter how old you are, it's never too soon or too late to take better care of yourself. And a great first step is to have a checkup with a doctor, midwife, or nurse who offers sexual or reproductive health care. These experts can support you in so many ways, like helping you:

- learn about how your body works, inside and out, and how to keep it clean and healthy.
- choose from menstrual (period) products or cope with period pain.

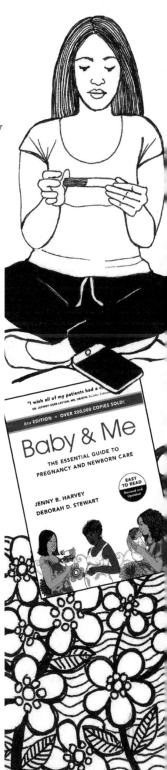

Look in this chapter for:

Track your periods. You can use an app or just mark off the days on a calendar. This helps you know when your cycle will start and also tells you if it is late.

- learn to track your period, so you know when to expect it and when it's late.

- figure out which feelings, smells, fluids, or pains are normal and which are not.

- talk through any worries or fears you have about sex or sexuality.

- learn about safe touch and consent, and how to get help if you are hurt or feel unsafe.

- create a plan for birth control or planning for pregnancy.

Many people get pregnant when they did not mean to. Most people don't know when they ovulate*, and many don't track their periods. Since sperm can live inside the uterus for up to five days after unprotected sex, it's not hard for a sperm to find your egg before you even miss a period. So many important things happen in the first months of pregnancy. Risky or unhealthy choices in these early weeks can cause problems that last baby's whole life. If there's any chance you could get pregnant, start taking care of your body now.

*__Ovulation:__ When an egg is released from an ovary and moves down the fallopian tube. This is when you are most fertile (likely to get pregnant).

- Tell your doctor or nurse if you think you might get pregnant. Ask if any health problems you have could make things hard. Ask if you should stop or change your medications while pregnant.

- Start using a type of birth control that works well (see chapter 16).

- Take a vitamin with folate (folic acid) in it every day.

- Stop using alcohol, tobacco, vape, pot, or other drugs. Don't stay in places where others are smoking or vaping.

- Take care of any health problems, such as diabetes or high blood pressure.

- Get health insurance if you don't have it already.

See chapters 3, 4, and 5 to learn more.

Fetal growth in the first two months (life size)

4 weeks

Cells for heart and brain start forming.

6 weeks (embryo)

Heart is beating, organs start forming, and neural tube is closing (will turn into brain, spinal cord, and spine.

8 weeks

Brain, face, and head grow. Arms grow finger buds, legs form, and parts of the eyes, ears, nose, and mouth can be seen. The placenta is working.

11 weeks (fetus)

Some organs start working, bones and tooth buds are forming, body takes shape. Genitals start forming.

Weeks are counted from the start of your last menstrual period (LMP).

Words for baby before birth: 0–10 weeks: *embryo*   11 weeks–birth: *fetus* Preterm

How do I know if I'm pregnant?

The first signs of pregnancy are:

- late period or no period.
- being tired.
- sore or swollen breasts.
- vomiting or nausea*.

*Nausea: The feeling of needing to vomit.

If your period is late and you have any of these signs, you might be pregnant. It's time for a pregnancy test. Start taking care of your body as if you were pregnant.

Pregnancy tests

Clinic or in-office tests can be done even before you miss a period. Many clinics, like Planned Parenthood, do them for free or low cost. These blood tests are very accurate. You may also have an ultrasound* if your period is more than a few weeks late.

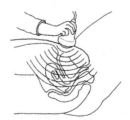 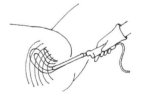

*Ultrasound: A way to see inside your body using sound waves. A special wand is placed on your belly or in your vagina to check your uterus and the fetus.

Home pregnancy tests can be bought at most markets or drug stores, with no prescription. These test your urine (pee) for certain hormones and can be used soon after your period should have started. A positive test result means you are pregnant. A negative test could mean you are not pregnant, or that you took it too soon. Wait a week and test again.

What do I do now?

Take extra care of your body right now. Look through this book. Think about your plans for starting a family. Read about how to take care of your body before and while you are pregnant.

If you are not pregnant

Think about what that means to you. You may be relieved, sad, or a bit of both.

If you are *glad* to not be pregnant, think about your birth control plan. See chapter 16 to learn about different types of birth control. You might talk to your provider to see if there is a better option for you. Use protection every single time you have sex.

If you are *sad* to not be pregnant, share your feelings with someone you trust. Talk with your partner about if and when you do want to have a baby. If that time comes, your provider can help you plan to get pregnant. See Chapters 3 and 4 to learn how to take good care of yourself as you prepare.

If you are pregnant

Parent support programs can help you feel ready to be a good parent. **See chapter 17 for more.**

Make an appointment with a doctor, nurse, or midwife. Tell them you are pregnant when you call. See chapters 3, 4, and 5 to learn more about being healthy and safe while pregnant.

If you are not sure you are ready to be a parent, talk to someone you trust right away. Share your worries with a doctor, nurse, counselor, social worker, or midwife. Or call your local Planned Parenthood or public health clinic. Ask what your options are and how long you have to decide. **Start on page 285 for where to learn more and get support as you decide.**

If you are ready to be a parent, your provider will likely want to see you one to two months after your first missed period. By that time, the baby is big enough to show on an ultrasound.

Now is the time to really think about what life will be like for you and your future baby. This book will help you explore what lies ahead.

Take a Breath

No matter what the future holds, it's important to take care of yourself. What you think and how you feel affects your whole body. Stress makes everything harder. What helps you relax?

- Slow, deep breaths. Close your eyes and relax your face. Breathe in as you count slowly to four, then pause. Breathe out as you count slowly to five. Do this five to ten times.

- Listen to music. Play something lively and have your own mini dance party. Or play something calm that feels soothing.

- Do some yoga or go for a walk with a friend. Moving your body can help you get rid of stress.

- Sit outside and have a cup of tea. Listen to the sounds around you. Fresh air and the sounds of nature can be very refreshing.

- Call a friend who you enjoy talking to. Someone you can laugh with or cry with. Feeling connected is good for you.

- Get cozy with a book or movie. Choose something that makes you laugh a lot. It's good for you!

- Eat a healthy snack or take a nap. Taking care of your body tells it that it's loved.

"I made a Chill Out Playlist that helps whenever I feel stressed."

"When I'm worried, I get under a blanket, turn on a funny movie, and knit. It works almost every time!"

What else helps you relax? _____

_____

_____

_____

_____

Crisis Pregnancy Centers (CPC) – BEWARE

There are places that *look* like a health clinic but are not licensed to provide medical services. Their ads may offer "help with unwanted pregnancies". They make it seem like they provide counseling or perform abortions. These are known as Crisis Pregnancy Centers. They are often faith-based and known to use shame, fear, and false information to stop people from getting abortions.

CPCs use lots of ads, signs, and billboards to lure people in. They are often found close to real sexual health clinics, like Planned Parenthood. If you make an appointment at a health or abortion clinic, be sure to ask for tips on how to find their entrance. If you get there but are unsure, call before you go inside to make sure you're in the right place. You deserve support and care you can trust.

The types of clinics recommended in this book provide safe, reliable education and health care based on your needs and decisions.

Who do I listen to?
Where do I find answers?

There are so many ways to get information these days. The internet, TV, podcasts, blogs, books, and billboards. People you know, even people you don't know! It can be really hard to know who to listen to and what to believe.

When it comes to your health or your baby's health, it's important to make sure you're getting good and true information. Major health and safety agencies and public health programs are the best places for lots of information. Your health care provider is also a good person to answer your questions. If you read or hear something you're not sure about, talk to your provider about it. If your provider seems wrong about something, ask another provider about it.

Chapter 17 has many resources you can trust.

This book was written using the most current information from health sources you can trust. It was also reviewed by many doctors, nurses, midwives, and other people with lots of training on these topics.

This is *your* body

Finding out that you're pregnant can be very overwhelming. If you didn't plan to get pregnant, it can feel like you're not in control. Your body is amazing and can do all kinds of things on its own! But you are still the one in charge.

The next chapter starts by talking about what it feels like to be pregnant, how to choose a provider, and what to expect at your prenatal checkups. **If you need to think through your options first, go to page 285 for a list of places that can help you while you decide what to do. Start at page 286 to learn more about your options. You can always come back here when you're ready.**

Learning about what is happening to your body right now is a great first step to feeling back in control. The next few chapters will give you the information you need to make the choices that are right for you.

Chapter 2

You're Pregnant— What's Next?

Being pregnant can make you feel both excited and scared. Most people have mixed feelings—and a lot of questions.

What is it like to give birth?

Will my baby be healthy?

Will I be a good parent?

How would a baby change my life?

It can be hard not knowing what life is going to be like later. Making some changes now can help make it easier down the road. Now is the time to learn about making a healthy life for you and baby.

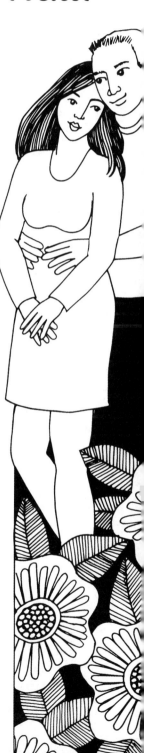

What's happening to me?

Your body starts to change in many ways before your belly starts to show. Some people feel different right away and others feel changes more slowly. You may have some cramps or spotting, but not a real period. You may feel bloated and sore in your belly and breasts as time goes on. Your energy level and moods may go up and down. You may feel like you need to vomit (throw up) or pee more often. The further into your pregnancy you get, the more changes you'll see.

How far along am I?

One of the first things you may want to know is how far along you are. A pregnancy is measured in weeks. A full pregnancy is 40 weeks long, including the weeks of your period and ovulation (when your ovaries release an egg). You can use an app to find out how many weeks along you are, or you can just use a calendar (see below).

Mark the day your last period started (we used "P"). Starting on this day, count the weeks until today's date. This is **how far along** you are in your pregnancy.

SUN	MON	TUE	WED	THU	FRI	SAT
		P	P	P	P	P
P	P	1				
		2				
		3				
		4				
		5				
	WEEK	6				

What if I know what day I got pregnant?

You might know what day you had sex or when a condom broke and assume that's when you got pregnant. Knowing when the sperm got into your body can give you an idea of about when you got pregnant, but not exactly when. Once inside the body, sperm can live for up to five days. And, most people don't know exactly when their egg is released. So, the sperm might not find an egg for almost a week after you have sex.

What if I don't know?

If you don't know when your last period started or when you had unprotected sex, tell your healthcare provider. They will do a pregnancy test (see chapter 1) to confirm you are pregnant and might do an ultrasound to measure how big the fetus is. This will help them decide how far along you are and when your due date is.

When will my baby be born?

You may also want to know when the baby will be born (due date). Your *estimated due date (EDD)* will be the day you are 40 weeks pregnant. **To find your EDD**, go back to that calendar and keep counting the weeks all the way up to 40. That date is your **due date**.

If this is your first baby, it's likely that labor will start around a week after your due date.

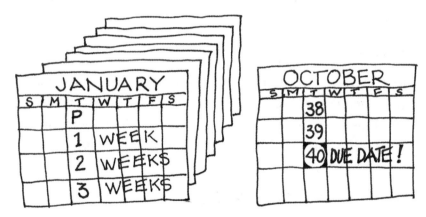

Words to describe babies at birth

Very few babies come on their exact due date. Most are born in the two weeks before or after. If all goes well, **labor will start when your baby and your body are ready.**

Babies who are born *at term* are usually developed well enough to be healthy outside the womb. Babies who are born preterm (very early) or postterm (very late) have higher risks of health problems. See page 175 for more on preterm babies.

Babies born:
Preterm (premature):
    born before 37 weeks
At term:
    37–38 weeks: *early term*
    39–40 weeks: *full term*
    41 weeks: *late term*
Postterm (post dates):
    born 42 weeks or more

Who do I call?

It can be hard to know where to start to find a new provider. Friends may have names of someone they like. Your insurance's help line can tell you who is on their list of providers. Or look up a public health clinic or Planned Parenthood. **If you don't have insurance**, these places, or the resources on page 288, can can help you sign up. See chapter 5 to learn about choosing care.

Get health care right away

Health care while you are pregnant is called **prenatal care**. Prenatal care is very important for both you and baby. You may be thrilled to be pregnant or scared that you're not ready to have a baby right now. No matter how you're feeling, **the next step is to go in for your first prenatal checkup**. If you don't want to see your normal doctor, or you don't have one, there are others who can help. Have your insurance card ready when you call and tell them you are pregnant.

Prenatal visits

Once you have your appointment set, you may feel excited and eager or nervous and scared. Take good care of yourself while you wait. Drink lots of water and get plenty of rest. You might ask someone who helps you feel safe and calm to come with you to your first appointment.

What will my first visit be like?

Your first prenatal visit will be the longest. Your provider will ask lots of questions about your health history and your family's health. They'll need to know what medicines or drugs you are taking. They'll ask when your last period started, when you had sex, and if you used any kind of birth control. They may ask if you have a safe place to live and people who support you. Be honest when you answer so they can offer help if you need it.

This is also your time to get to know your provider. Ask questions. Tell them what fears or concerns you have. Ask what to expect at your visits and ask them to explain what they're going to do. Tell them if you are uncomfortable or need a break.

They will also do a full physical exam. It will likely include:

- checking your blood pressure, height, and weight.
- a breast exam: your provider looks at and feels your breasts and armpits for signs of problems.
- a pelvic exam*: an internal exam to check your uterus, ovaries, and fallopian tubes.

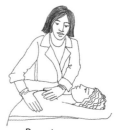

Breast exam

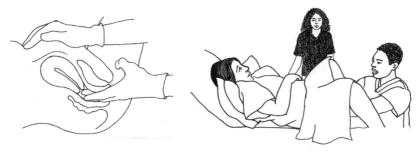

***Pelvic exam:** Your provider places their gloved fingers inside your vagina. Their other hand gently presses on the outside of your lower belly.*

- Pap, HPV, or STI* tests: during your pelvic exam, your provider may gently wipe cells or fluid from your cervix to check for disease or infection. Your provider will use a tool (**speculum**) to hold your vagina open so they can see your cervix.
- blood or urine samples to check blood type and screen for diabetes, anemia, and certain diseases.
- talking about what vaccines to get while pregnant.

***STI (or STD):** A sexually transmitted infection or disease.*

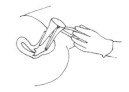

Your provider will use a tool (**speculum**) to hold your vagina open so they can see your cervix.

Depending on how far along you might be, they may use an ultrasound to look for and measure your fetus. Using the date of your last period and how big the fetus is, your provider will figure out your due date.

See chapter 5 to learn more about tests, ultrasounds, and what else to expect at your checkups.

When to talk to your provider*

It's important to be able to talk to your provider if you are worried. Ask what the best way to get in touch with them is between checkups. If you have pain or any of the **warning signs on page 94,** it is best to call. They may have a number to call on nights and weekends to reach them quickly. If it feels less urgent, you might just send a message in their "patient portal" or "chat

***Provider:** The doctor, nurse, or midwife who gives you health care.*

with a provider" on their website or app. Put all of these numbers and links into your phone or computer so it's easy to find them.

Your provider will need you to tell them what is going on. What is your temperature, how you are feeling, and how long has it been that way? Has it felt the same or is it getting worse? Be honest so they can know how to help you. Write down what they say to do or watch out for.

Who can give you support?

Finding out you are pregnant can bring up big feelings. It is important for you to have someone in your life who will help you feel safe and cared for. No matter what you decide or how this pregnancy goes, you deserve comfort and support.

In this book, we talk about partners a lot. Partners are an important part of pregnancy, birth, and being a parent. Who that partner is, though, is whoever is right for you. It might be one person or it might be a group of people.

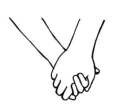

This book has partner tips at the end of each chapter. Many of these tips will help anyone know how to support you, but some are mainly for a romantic partner. Take a look as you read and see what you'd like to share with whoever is going through this with you.

Your romantic partner

If you got pregnant by someone you are in a caring relationship with, it may be good to tell them early on. Talk to them about how you're feeling, good or bad. Ask them how they're feeling, too. Partners play a big role in a healthy pregnancy. You are the one in charge of your body, but it is still nice to know that they are on your side.

If you got pregnant by having sex with someone you aren't in a relationship with, think about if they would be a good support to you. Do you trust them and feel safe telling them you're pregnant? If so, it may help to talk to them and let them support you, no matter what you decide.

If you don't have a partner

You don't have to go through this alone. Close friends and family can be great support during pregnancy and birth. Find a few people who you can count on to listen and help you feel safe and loved. Some health clinics have support groups or prenatal classes for single parents.

You'll also want to take some time to think about who will be with you when your baby is born. Maybe a family member or a friend. You could also find out about low-cost doulas* in your area. Having support during pregnancy, birth, and after is very important.

*Doula: A person trained to give comfort and support to you before, during, and after birth. Not a medical professional but often very helpful.

Your family

Some families are more able to offer support than others. Parents, aunts or uncles, grandparents, or even older siblings or cousins. Having family beside you, even in those first weeks or months, can really help. If your family can't support you, look to your friends or community.

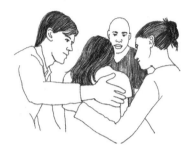

Your friends

Sometimes it's easier to talk to a good friend about big things like this. Especially if you're scared or unsure. Think about friends who you really trust and who have been there for you when you've needed them. Maybe you have a friend whose family you trust and feel close to. The more caring people you have around you, the better.

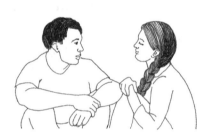

Your community

There are a lot of ways to get support, even from people you don't know yet! If you go to school or a place of worship, they might know of a group or program that could help. Your local family center, health clinic, human services office, or Planned Parenthood may have support for people in your situation. You might find all kinds of things, from support groups to walking meet-ups!

Many online groups offer a place to connect with people, too. Look for groups that share your interests or that have things in common with you. It's a good idea to find a group that has ground rules for making sure it's a safe space.

Don't share your full name or address online.

Talking about sex or pregnancy can be awkward or embarrassing. Still, you might be surprised by how many people care and want to help. There are so many ways people can offer support, now and later. It could be a hand to hold, a meal to share, or a ride to your appointment.

*If you don't have safe people in your life, **see chapter 17 for where to get support by phone, text, or online.***

Sharing your news

Talking to your partner

Telling your partner you are pregnant may feel scary. But waiting a long time to tell them can be hard on both of you.

You may feel it's best to tell them early on. That way, you aren't alone when you find out for sure if you're pregnant or not. They can come to your first prenatal visit and help talk through what happens next.

You may want to get the facts and decide what to do before telling your partner. This may feel like the best option for people who don't think their partner will react well to the news. If you're not sure, talk to someone else you trust first. Practice what you might say and ask if you can call them if you need some support afterwards.

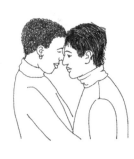

When you do tell your partner, do it in a place where you feel safe and comfortable. Make sure you have lots of time to really talk and be there for each other. If you've already decided what to do next, tell them. If you're still not sure, share your worries. Think about how you'd like your partner to help. You may both have mixed feelings and need time to sort it out. Your pregnancy is going to be a big deal for them, too. Be patient with yourself and each other.

If you do not feel safe talking to your partner, ask someone else you trust for help.

Talking to your family

For some people, telling their parents or family that they're pregnant is exciting. For others, it can be overwhelming and hard. There are many reasons you might worry about your family's reaction to the news. Maybe you are very young, or not in a good

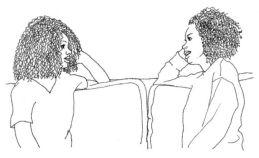

relationship, or don't have a job. Or maybe they don't believe in sex before marriage, or you just don't want to disappoint them.

Think first about what you will say. Do you want to see a doctor first? Do you want to decide what to do before you tell them? Do you want your partner, a friend, or someone else to be there with you?

They may be shocked when you tell them. They might be upset and yell or cry at first. They may need some time to let the news sink in. But most parents and relatives really do want to support their kids and family members when they get pregnant. They want to help them be safe and healthy, even if that means helping with a baby.

Keep in mind that it won't just be one talk and then done. No matter what happens with your pregnancy, you will have a lot of feelings and decisions in the coming months. And your family probably will, too. Try to be patient and honest with yourself and your family.

If you do not feel safe talking to your family, ask someone else you trust for help. See chapter 17 for support programs.

Your partner's family may also need to be told, especially if you are very young. Talk to your partner about how they feel about telling their family. Maybe you want your family to come with you, or maybe you want to tell them all together. Even if your partner is not supportive, their family might want to help.

Hey, partner!

This book is for you, too! Even if this is the first time you've really thought about pregnancy and babies, this book will help you make sense of it all.

Look for the image of the holding hands at the end of each chapter. That's where you'll find tips that are just for you! It may be things to think about, how to help your partner, or what to plan for in the coming months.

Be sure to check out the glossary and resources in the back of the book for more information.

If you do not have a supportive partner, think of who else might give you the support you need. When you see Tips for Partners at the end of each chapter, who could help you in those ways? You can do this and you're not alone. Ask your provider about a health advocate or low-cost doula.

Mixed feelings

Both you and your partner may have mixed feelings about being pregnant and what comes next. That is normal and ok! Take some time to think through your thoughts and feelings below:

Practice taking a long deep breath if you are stressed

(Check how you feel)

_____ It's wonderful.

_____ It feels strange.

_____ It's hard to believe.

_____ I don't feel ready to have a baby.

(write your own)

I am happy about _____

I wonder about _____

I am worried about _____

I need help _____

When you are ready, show this to your partner and ask them to share their thoughts. Even if you don't feel the same, try to be open with each other. Remind yourselves that you're on the same team.

Tips for partners

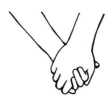

Getting pregnant will change your life, too. There are many ways to be a good partner, right from the start.

- ◆ Ask your partner how they feel about being pregnant. Listen patiently while they answer.
- ◆ Ask if they have decided on next steps.
- ◆ Share how you are feeling about the pregnancy and what happens next.

- Offer to help talk through these hard choices, but remember that it is your partner's body.
- Offer your love and support. You'll both have lots of feelings, so try to be gentle and kind.
- Talk together about planning for the future.

Chapter 3

Keeping Your Body Healthy

What you do every day is important for your baby's health—and your own. It's easy to say, "live a healthy life." But, do you know what that means and how to do it? This chapter can help.

Now that you are pregnant, you have the best reason in the world for changing your habits. These habits are good for everyone. But, they are more important than ever during pregnancy.

I feel fine, so why do I need so many checkups?

Prenatal care is medical care for your pregnancy. You will have a lot of prenatal visits. These checkups help your health care provider learn how your baby and you are doing. They will look for health problems you can't feel.

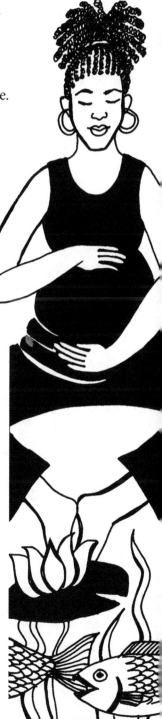

If you and baby are both doing well, you will have one visit each month. In the last two months, you will have more checkups. Your provider will check:

- your baby's growth, heart rate, and movement.
- how you feel and how your body is changing.
- how much weight you've gained.
- your blood pressure*.
- any chronic health issues that may affect your pregnancy.

*Blood pressure:
The force of the blood pumped by the heart through your blood vessels. High blood pressure means the heart is working extra hard.

Most people have healthy babies. Regular visits help make this happen. Checkups can help catch problems early. Early treatment of any problems is best.

Your provider wants to hear your questions. What are you worried about? What do you want to know more about? Your prenatal visits are the best time to ask questions. As you go through this book, write down questions that you want to ask on the checkup pages. These are in chapters 7, 8, and 9.

For more about prenatal visits and finding a provider, see chapter 5.

Healthy habits

Your health care provider is your best first source of information. But, there are many sources of health advice, like books, TV shows, websites, or people you know. Some of what you hear or read may not be true.

Some advice can be very confusing. You may hear good news one day about a product, food, or activity. The next day, some other source may say it is not healthy. Which advice can you believe?

You are making a good start by using this book. It has been written using the newest information from health sources you can trust. Doctors, nurses, midwives, and others with proper training have reviewed it.

Here are questions to ask before you trust something new that you hear or read:

- Where did the information first come from (person, company, or organization)? Is it a source that you can trust? You can trust the national health organizations listed in chapter 17.

- Are they trying to sell something?

- Is the report new? Look for a date on books or pamphlets. Some may be so old that they are out of date. But, news on TV or the web may be so new that it hasn't really been proven.

- Have you asked your doctor or midwife about the advice you've heard? What do they tell you?

Start healthy habits right now

The baby inside you is growing fast. Look back at the pictures of the very tiny baby in chapter 1. All the main parts of the body (brain, spinal cord, and organs) are formed in the first two months. This is why you need to take care of yourself from the start of pregnancy.

Life-size pictures

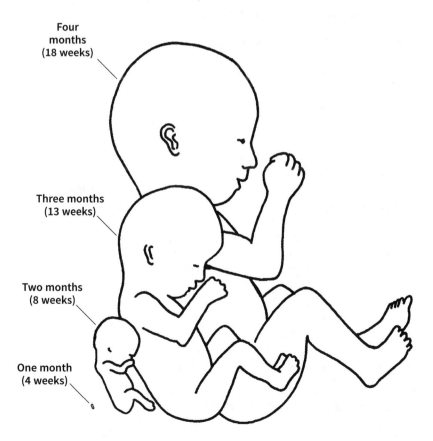

Four months (18 weeks)

Three months (13 weeks)

Two months (8 weeks)

One month (4 weeks)

The pictures on page 23 show how much your baby grows in the first four months. Even more amazing changes are taking place inside!

What are healthy habits?

Most of us have at least a few bad habits. Some may not be a big deal, but others can put both you and baby at serious risk. Making healthy choices gets easier the more we do it.

How are you doing right now?

It's good to check in with yourself often. Feel proud of the good things you are already doing. Set goals for what you would like to change. Try to be honest as you fill out the chart below.

Nobody's perfect, but you are making a good start!

Healthy Habits	Yes	Some-times	No
I drink 8–12 glasses of water each day			
I eat at least 5 servings of fruit & veggies a day			
I sleep at least 7–8 hours each night			
I'm active for at least 30 minutes most days			
I talk about my worries with others			
I have safe sex and only have one partner			
I brush and floss my teeth each day			
Unhealthy Habits	**Yes**	**Some-times**	**No**
I sit for more than 6 hours straight each day			
I drink beer, wine, hard seltzer, or liquor			
I smoke or chew tobacco			
I vape or use e-cigarettes			
I use illegal drugs or prescription drugs not from my doctor			
I have unprotected sex or have many partners			
I use marijuana or cannabis products			

What do you want to change? Write some ideas here:

_____

_____

_____

_____

Don't be afraid to ask for help. Making changes is not always easy, but it is worth it for baby! See chapter 17 for resources.

Making changes is easier when you do it together. Flip to page 40 to have your partner fill out the same questions. Then you can set goals together!

Get care for health problems

Your body is your baby's home right now. Your health and wellness affect baby. Pregnancy can bring a lot of joy, but it is also very demanding. Making sure you are well can give you the energy to look forward to the changes ahead.

- ◆ If you have a disease, illness, or injury, see a doctor now.
- ◆ If you have a hard time coping with stress, handling your feelings, or being kind to your body, find a therapist or counselor.
- ◆ If you don't have health insurance, call or visit your school nurse or local public health clinic. Ask for help signing up for state insurance.

Take care of teeth and gums

Good oral health is important while pregnant. Tooth and gum problems are more common in pregnancy. These problems can cause infections that may lead to baby being very small or born too soon. If you have those germs in your mouth, they can pass to baby after birth and put their tiny teeth at risk.

"My dentist said that my tooth problems can cause my baby problems that last for years! Now I have a note on my mirror so I don't forget to brush and floss."

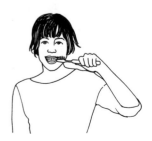

What can I do?

Brush and floss!

Brush your teeth for two minutes, twice a day. Use a soft toothbrush if your gums bleed.

Floss your teeth well, once a day.

Go to the dentist

Have a checkup with your dentist. Tell them you are pregnant.
Go in right away if you have any of these problems:

- Gums that bleed easily
- Bad breath that won't go away
- Sores or lumps in your mouth
- A loose or sore tooth

Your dentist can help you get your mouth healed before baby
is born.

If you do not have a dentist, ask your provider or insurance
company how to find one.

Stay active

Being active is good for both you and baby. Exercise helps you get
stronger, sleep better, and feel happier. It can also help you:

- stay at a healthy weight during and after pregnancy.
- keep blood sugar and blood pressure normal.
- lower the chance of labor starting too early.
- lessen back aches, hip pain, stiffness, swelling, and varicose veins*.
- help with gas, constipation, and hemorrhoids*.

*Varicose veins:
Swollen blue veins in
your legs that can

*Hemorrhoids:
Swollen veins in your
bottom (anus) that
may itch, bleed, or be
sore.

What kinds of exercise are best?

Talk with your provider about what kinds of exercise they advise.
If you don't already exercise, start with something easy like
walking. Try to be active for 30 minutes at least three or four
times a week.

- Most activites are safe to keep doing while pregnant, but not all. Try to avoid things that are very bouncy. Don't do things that could make you fall, jump, or get hit in the belly.
- Walking is one of the best exercises. It is good for your whole body. And, it's easy and free! Wear good walking shoes and bring a water bottle.
- Swimming is great during pregnancy. It's good for your heart and helps calm swelling. Feeling so light in the water can also feel very good.

- Exercise and gently stretch the core* of your body. This will help lessen back aches during pregnancy. It will make you strong for pushing in childbirth. You may be more flexible than normal, so be careful not to go too far.

- Prenatal yoga is good for your core. It also helps you learn to relax. This will be very helpful when you are in labor.

- Don't fall! Your balance changes and makes falls more common while pregnant. See page 39 for how to avoid falls

*Core: Your tummy (abs) and back muscles.

Ways to make exercising easier

- Walk with a friend. Exercising together, you can get each other moving. It can make exercise less boring.

- You can exercise for 10 or 15 minutes a few times a day. This can be easier for you than one longer session.

- Try an exercise class. Many hospitals, gyms, and community centers offer prenatal classes. Look for a walking or swimming group for pregnant people in your area.

What else should I know about exercise?

- Drink plenty of water before, during, and after exercise.
- Exercise when it's cool outside. Try not to get too hot.
- Be extra careful if you live in high altitude, or where it gets very hot or very cold.
- Sit down and rest if you are uncomfortable, dizzy, too hot, or have trouble breathing.

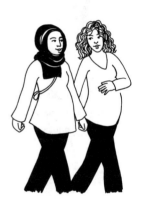

"I hate exercising. But when my friend and I started walking together, the time just flew by! It got me out the door twice a week and we talked about all kinds of things."

STOP exercising and call your provider if you:

- Get dizzy or lightheaded often
- Have pain in your chest, belly, or legs
- Get a headache or have trouble seeing
- Have sudden swelling in your legs
- Feel sudden tightness or squeezing across your belly (contractions)
- Have blood or fluid coming from your vagina

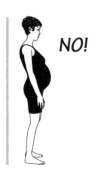

NO!

Does your back curve and belly hang out? This is a habit you can break.

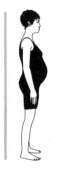

Get in the habit of standing straight and pulling in your belly.

Great exercises for your core (tummy and back)

Start strengthening your tummy and back right away. Many people don't do this before pregnancy, so their muscles need a lot of work. You can do these simple exercises when you are standing, sitting, or lying in bed.

Standing tall and straight Standing with your belly hanging forward can make your back hurt. Standing up straight can lessen low-back pain. Walking straight also helps you feel good about yourself. Watch yourself do it in a big mirror the first time.

1. Wear comfortable shoes with a low heel. Stand sideways to the mirror. See how curved your low back is.
2. Now, pull your chin down and keep your ears right above your shoulders.
3. Take a deep breath and pull your shoulders back. Squeeze your shoulder blades down your back.
4. Let your breath out. Pull your tummy in. Keep your shoulders back. Check to see that your lower back is less curved.
5. Move back and forth a few times to get the feel for it.

See how your body looks different. Feel how your tummy and back muscles work together. Practice standing and walking this way. It will be good for you now and after baby comes, too.

One way to practice is to stand with your back to the wall and pull your back and shoulders back against the wall.

"Pelvic tilt" helps back pain This makes your stomach muscles stronger and stretches your back. It can help you carry the extra weight without hurting your back.

1. Rest on hands and knees with your back straight.
2. Breathe in and pull your shoulders back. Lift your chest. Hold and count to five.
3. Breathe out while you tighten your tummy muscles. Pull your shoulders forward and arch your back like a cat.
4. Hold and count to five.
5. Breathe in again and pull your shoulders back. Flatten your back.

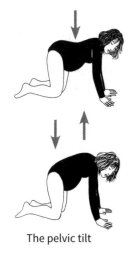

The pelvic tilt

After the first four months, do this standing up.

Arm and leg lifts Use this exercise to strengthen your back.

1. Rest on hands and knees with your back straight. Pull in your belly.
2. Raise one arm straight out. Then raise the opposite leg straight out.
3. Hold and count to five.
4. Lower the arm and leg.
5. Raise the other arm and opposite leg. Count to five.
6. Repeat 10 times on each side.

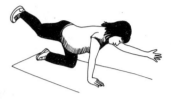

Arm and leg lift

Drink water and carry snacks

Water is very important for all parts of your body. While pregnant, try to drink 8 to 12 glasses (80 to 96 ounces) each day. You will need more water in hot weather, after exercise, if you have a fever, and if you vomit or have diarrhea. Getting enough water helps with blood flow, constipation, swelling, and urinary tract infections. Try to bring water with you wherever you go.

It is also a good idea to bring healthy snacks with you. Nuts, dried fruit, and granola bars are all easy to put in your bag for when you need a burst of energy. Having healthy snacks at home is also important. Fruit, vegetables, cheese, boiled eggs, yogurt, nut butter on toast, or hummus with crackers are all quick and healthy snacks between meals. See chapter 4 for more on healthy eating.

Get enough rest

One of the first things you notice about being pregnant is being very tired. Most pregnant women need 8 to 10 hours of sleep each day. If you can't get enough sleep at night, try to take naps during the day. Make sleep a priority now because it gets harder later in pregnancy.

Stay safe on the road

Getting out is good for you. Being active and getting fresh air and exercise. Having fun with friends and family. Going to work or school. And don't forget all of those prenatal checkups you'll be having! Be safe on the go to protect both you and baby.

Driving or riding in a vehicle is likely the most risky thing you'll do each day.

Do you ride safely? (Check the things you always do.)

_____ I always use a seat belt, even in the back seat. If the bus has seat belts, I use them.

_____ I drive a car that has airbags.

_____ I say "no" to riding with a driver who has been drinking or using drugs.

_____ If I need to text or answer a phone call, I stop the car first. I know both are distracting and often cause crashes.

Buckle up!

Most people who are hurt or killed in car crashes weren't wearing a seat belt. Seat belts and airbags work together to keep you from slamming into things or being thrown out of the car. But, it's important to use them properly.

Getting your seat belt to fit right can be tricky while pregnant. The lap belt may creep up on your belly and the shoulder belt may slide up onto your neck. It's very important to keep the seatbelt in the right position.

The best seat belt

Whenever possible, use a lap-shoulder seat belt. This is the kind that goes across your lap and up over your shoulder. These protect you much more than a lap-only belt. After you sit down and buckle:

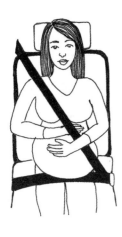

- slide the lap belt under your belly, on the tops of your thighs.
- place the shoulder belt across your chest, between your breasts.
- pull up on the shoulder belt to get the whole seat belt snug.
- make sure the shoulder belt goes over your collar bone, not up on your neck or off your shoulder.
- if the car you're in has an adjuster for how high the shoulder belt is, move it down so the shoulder belt is close to your shoulder, but not below it.

Where and how to sit

As baby grows, so does your belly. Your belly is sort of like your baby's first car seat. If you go flying and get hurt, so does baby. The safest place to sit is in a seat that has a lap-shoulder belt that fits you well. If you can, adjust the bottom of the seat higher. This can help the lap belt stay down off the belly.

Keep your seat back more upright to help the seatbelt fit well. This is safer in a crash. Unless your belly is too close to the steering wheel, try not to recline your seat.

"As my belly got bigger, it kept getting closer to my steering wheel! The doctor said it's safer to let someone else drive whenever I can."

Move your seat back as far as you can. This gives your belly more space so it's less likely to slam into anything. Airbags are helpful, but you don't want to be too close if it bursts out in a crash. Try to keep your belly at least 10 inches away from the steering wheel, dashboard, or frontal airbag.

What about airbags?

All newer cars today have at least two front airbags, one in the steering wheel and another in the dashboard. A front airbag works *with* the seat belt to protect you in a crash. It does not replace the seat belt. You still need the seat belt to protect you and keep you in the car.

How to sit safely in a car with air bags:

+ Sit back from the dashboard or steering wheel. Move your seat as far back as it can go.

+ Keep your belly and chest at least 10 inches away from the dash or steering wheel, if you can.

+ If your steering wheel tilts, aim it at your chest, not your head or belly.

+ If you have a hard time reaching the pedals, try reclining the back. Then move the seat forward.

Most newer cars have side airbags, too. These may be in the doors, walls, or seats. Some seat belts also have airbags in the shoulder part. Check the car owner's manual for advice.

When it's not safe to drive

It's usually okay to drive during pregnancy. But, sometimes it's dangerous. Being very tired or feeling sick can make it hard to focus on driving. Even just having a lot on your mind can make you distracted.

Don't drive if you are dizzy, have a headache, or have vision problems. It's better not to drive if you don't have to.

If you are in a crash

Get checked out at an emergency room or doctor's office right away after any kind of crash. Do this even if you feel okay.

Be sure to tell the doctor you are pregnant. It's important to make sure your baby, uterus, placenta, and the rest of your body aren't hurt.

Baby will need a car seat

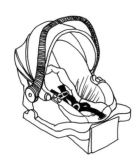

Right now your body and your seat belt protect your baby. But, they will need their own car seat (child safety seat) after birth. You will need to use it for every car ride. Car seats protect babies very well and are required by law in all states. (See chapter 6 for how to choose a car seat. Read chapter 14 for how to use it right.)

Have safe sex

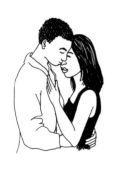

Some parts of your body can feel very sensitive while pregnant. This may mean that sex feels great to you and you want to have a lot of it. Or, this may mean it's uncomfortable and you don't want to have as much. Listen to your body and do what feels good to you. Talk to your provider if sex is painful or not working well for you.

*Miscarriage** is when baby dies before your 20th week of pregnancy. See page 99 for more.

Just because you're already pregnant doesn't mean unprotected sex is safe. You can still get sexually transmitted infections (STIs) from any kind of sexual contact. STIs can be very harmful to a growing fetus and can even cause miscarriage.* If you think you may have an STI, be sure to say so when you go in for your checkup. Most STIs can be treated during pregnancy. Some can't be cured, but treatment can keep them from spreading to baby. If you have sex, use a condom every time. Or make sure you and your partner both test negative for STIs and aren't having sex with any other people. See chapter 8 for more about sex during pregnancy.

Stop dangerous habits

Anything you put into your body can also go into baby's body. Drugs, cigarettes, nicotine, and alcohol are very dangerous for baby. They can cause lifelong problems for baby and even lead to premature birth, miscarriage, or stillbirth*. There are many ways to get help quitting these habits. Talk to your provider or your local public health program to find help. See chapter 4 to learn more.

*Stillbirth is when a baby who dies before or during birth from 20 weeks on is called stillborn.

Germs and your unborn baby

It is never fun to get sick. But, getting sick while pregnant can be very hard and even dangerous for baby.

Easy ways to prevent sickness

People in good health get sick less than people who don't take care of themselves. Take care of yourself in all the ways talked about in this book. Also:

1. Avoid people who seem sick.
2. Wash hands often.
3. Get your **vaccines**. Get your flu, COVID, and TdAP (whooping cough) shots. Talk to your provider about other vaccines you may want while you are pregnant.
4. Have those around you get their vaccines, too. This helps keep baby safe after birth, too.

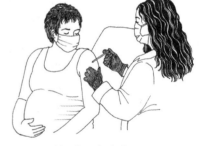

Vaccines help keep you and your baby safe from dangerous illness.

If you do get sick

Ask your provider what kinds of symptoms you should call for. Watch out for fever, dehydration, rashes, or signs of infection. Ask your provider before taking any kind of medicine. Some medicines are not safe to take while pregnant.

Germs to watch out for
Influenza (FLU)

Flu is a common viral illness. It can cause a fever, cough, sore throat, runny or stuffy nose, chills, and head or body aches. Flu can be mild, but pregnant people are more likely to get very sick from it. It can also put baby at risk of preterm birth. Flu is spread in droplets (tiny drops of fluid) that come from an infected person's mouth or nose with they laugh, cough, sneeze, or talk. It is most common to catch it when you breathe in these droplets, but it can also spread if you touch something that the droplets have landed on.

How can I protect myself and baby? There are tests and medicines for the flu that can help keep it mild if you see a doctor as soon as you think you are sick. Get your vaccine! Flu shots are safe while pregnant and can help keep your illness very mild.

Coronavirus (SARS-CoV-2 or "COVID-19")

"Even though we don't have to wear masks in town anymore, I still wear one on the bus and in waiting rooms."

COVID-19 is a virus that causes flu-like symptoms and is spread very easily. It can be mild for some, but very dangerous for others. Pregnant people who get COVID-19 are more likely to get very sick. While it is very rare to pass COVID-19 to your unborn baby, it does increase the risk of preterm birth or stillbirth.

How can I protect myself and baby? The best thing you can do is get your COVID-19 vaccines. Talk to your provider about getting your vaccine while pregnant and plan for baby to have one when they are old enough. (Ask baby's provider when they can get their first COVID vaccine.) Wash your hands often and use a hand sanitizer (with alcohol) when you can't. Wear a well-fitted face mask in crowded places or around people who might be sick. Ask friends and family to wear a mask or take COVID-19 tests before visiting.

*CDC: Centers for Disease Control www.cdc.gov

COVID rates go up and down quickly. Check the CDC* or your local health department for the current guidelines.

Respiratory Syncytial Virus (RSV)

RSV is a common virus that has symptoms like a common cold. While it's most often mild for adults, RSV is the leading reason babies are hospitalized in the US.

How can I protect my baby? If you are 32–36 weeks pregnant during the Fall or Winter, you can get a dose of RSV vaccine. Getting the vaccine this late in pregnancy means that baby is protected by those antibodies when they are born.

Babies born just before or during RSV season whose birth parent did not get the vaccine in pregnancy, they get their own vaccine. Talk to your provider about the best option for you and your baby.

There's a vaccine for that!

Vaccines work by helping your body make antibodies* for certain germs. They prepare your body for fighting off that sickness. This means you don't get sick at all or, if you do, your symptoms are much more mild.

*__Antibodies__: Special cells that find and attack germs.

What vaccines should I get while I'm pregnant?

Some vaccines are very safe for pregnant people and their unborn babies. Getting vaccines during pregnancy can even pass some protection on to baby! Getting your **flu, Tdap (whooping cough), RSV,** and **COVID-19** vaccines while pregnant will help your body make those antibodies. Some of those antibodies will go through your blood and into baby.

Are there vaccines I shouldn't get while pregnant?

Some vaccines are not safe to get during pregnancy. For example, measles and chicken pox are both risky for an unborn baby, but so are the vaccines. The best protection is to plan ahead and get up to date on your own vaccines before you get pregnant. Talk to your provider about getting your vaccine records. Tell them if you plan to travel while you try to get pregnant and ask about other vaccines that you may need.

Pertussis (whooping cough)

Whooping cough can be severe for anyone, but it can be deadly for a newborn, especially in the first two months.

How can I protect myself and baby? Getting a **Tdap** vaccine while pregnant passes antibodies to baby. The best time to get it is between 27 and 36 weeks. This gives baby's body time to build up enough protection to stay healthy right after birth. Then they can get their own vaccine at two months.

Zika

Zika virus is often very mild for adults. But, it can cause very severe birth defects in unborn babies. It is mostly spread by mosquito bites in places that have Zika, like Central and South America. It can also be spread by having sex without a condom with someone who has the virus.

How can I protect myself and baby? There is no medicine or vaccine for Zika. It is safest to avoid places with Zika. If you can't, then wear long sleeves and insect repellent (spray) to keep mosquitos away.

Cytomegalovirus (CMV)

CMV virus can pass to baby during pregnancy and can cause birth defects and hearing loss. It is often spread through the saliva and urine of young children.

How can I protect myself and baby? There is no vaccine for CMV. You can lessen your risk by washing hands after changing diapers and not sharing food and drink with children.

Germs carried by pets and animals

Cat poop has germs in it that can cause birth defects in an unborn baby even if you don't feel sick. Chickens, turtles, and other animals can also carry harmful germs. If you can, have someone else clean up after your pets while you're pregnant. If you must do it yourself, wear gloves and wash your hands well afterwards. If you have mice or rats in your home, have your landlord or someone else get rid of them safely.

Take a look around you

Simple habits like washing your hands, taking off your shoes at the door, and using a water filter can protect you and baby against many risks. But, there are still many things to watch out for.

Poisonous chemicals

Many chemicals are risky for an unborn baby. Some chemicals have a strong smell and are easy to notice, others give you no clues that they're there.

Do not use a generator, barbeque, or fire pit indoors. Even a kitchen oven can cause toxic fumes and lead to fires if used to heat the home.

- Cleaning products: try to use natural cleaners instead of harsh chemicals or bleach. Wear gloves.
- Fumes: open windows while cleaning. Use kitchen fans while cooking or to clear smells. Get fresh air into the house if you paint or get new carpet, furniture, or baby gear.

- Smoke and vape: stay away from cigarette smoke and people using e-cigarettes or vape pens.

- Pests: avoid using bug spray or other poisons in or around your home.

- Body care: use soaps, lotions, and sunscreens that have fewer chemicals and fragrances.

- Plastics: try to use plastic food containers that are BPA free. Avoid putting plastic in the microwave.

Lead

Lead (pronounced "led") is a dangerous poison. Eating or breathing even a very small amount can cause miscarriage. It can lead to serious brain damage to unborn babies and young children. Lead can be found in the air, water, or dirt. It is in some paints, plastic, and metal. Some dishes, jewelry, makeup, and toys have lead in them, too. Buildings built before 1978 may have more lead in their walls and pipes. People who work jobs like painting, plumbing, construction, car repair, or handling batteries are most likely to breathe or ingest lead dust or track it into the house.

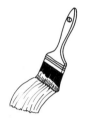

Lead is very bad for babies and kids. Get rid of it before baby is born.

How can I protect myself and baby?

If you think your home may have lead, tell your landlord you want a lead assessment. Each state has programs to make sure proper lead tests are done. Call the National Lead Information Center at 800-424-5323.

Learn more about how to protect your family from lead at *www.epa. gov/lead*

The most common sources of lead in homes:

- Old paint

- If it is not chipped or peeling, you can paint over it with a lead-free paint. Do not sand or scrape it first. Damaged paint should be removed and repainted while you are out of the house.

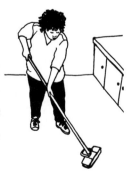

- Dirt and dust—Wash hands with soap after being outside. Use a nail brush if you've been gardening or cleaning. Have everyone take their shoes off when they come in the house. Wipe, mop, or vacuum window sills, floors, and other surfaces often.

If you are worried about your tap water, call the EPA Drinking Water Hotline at **800-426-4791** or visit **www.epa.gov /ground-water-and -drinking-water**

◆ Tap water—use cold water for cooking and drinking. Run faucet for 15–30 seconds before using water. Call your local public health department or water company to request lead testing.

Mercury

Mercury can cause damage to an unborn baby's brain, spine, lungs, and other organs. Mercury is found in glass thermometers and light bulbs. If these break, have someone else clean it up safely and throw it away. Some batteries, old clocks, and even some face creams have mercury in them.

Some kinds of fish have a lot of mercury in them, too. Fish is a healthy food in pregnancy, but it is important to avoid those high in mercury. See chapter 4 for more on choosing fish.

Wildfire smoke

Check *airnow.gov* for air quality reports. Follow "sensitive individuals" guidelines.

Clean air is always the best, especially while pregnant. Try to stay away from smoke of any kind while pregnant. During wildfire season, check the air quality in your area before going outside. Even if you can't smell the smoke, the air could still have harmful ash or chemicals in it. Follow your local public health agency's guidelines for keeping the air inside your home fresh and cool. Fans, air filters, and blocking outside air can help a lot.

If you have to go outside, an N-95 mask will work well, but cloth masks don't keep out tiny bits of smoke dust.

Heating up: Hot tubs and more

Getting too hot is not good for baby. Avoid hot yoga, sunbathing, or saunas. Only use a hot tub if the water is cooler than 100°F (37.8°C). Stick with warm baths and showers.

Fall risks

The next most common way pregnant people get seriously hurt is by falling. Falls are risky for everyone, but right now falls can hurt both you and your unborn baby.

Why are falls so common while pregnant?

Your growing belly can really change your balance. Swelling or joint pain may make it easy to slip or step wrong. As your belly grows, it makes it hard to see things that might trip you.

What can I do?

Staying active can help your balance keep up with your changing body. It can also help your muscles stay strong and protect your joints. Using a pregnancy support belt* can also help keep your body lined up for good balance.

*Support belt: A strap or band that snugly wraps around the back or hips. It can help support a heavy belly or painful back or pelvis.

Many pregnant people get dizzy when they get up too quickly. This can make it easy to fall, too. Make sure you drink plenty of water and eat often. Take a moment to find your balance when you stand up after sitting or lying down.

Falls are a huge danger people of all ages. (They're also the most common cause of injury in babies!) Now is a great time to make your home and habits as low risk as you can. Get rid of tripping hazards, like rugs that slide or cords across the floor. Use handrails on stairs. Put a non-slip mat in the bathroom. Make more trips instead of carrying large piles of stuff or heavy bags.

On the job risks

Working around heat, toxins, or machinery can be dangerous. So can heavy lifting, pulling, or working in places where you might fall. Even caregiving can be risky with diapers, body fluids, x-rays, or fumes. If your job has any of these risks, talk to your provider. You might ask your boss if there is a different job you can do while you're pregnant and nursing.

Even low-risk jobs can make problems worse in pregnancy. Sitting or standing in one place all day can cause swelling and stiffness. Long hours or not having enough breaks can be very stressful. Talk to your supervisor about taking breaks to stretch, put your feet up, or take a quick walk a few times a day.

"Wearing flat shoes and support socks really helped me get though my work day!"

If you are having serious health problems, ask your boss if you can do work that's less hard while you are pregnant. If they say no, you may be able to get a leave of absence or go on disability.

Tips for partners

It can be hard to know how to ask for help. They might not even know what they need yet! Now is the time to start really thinking about how to support them. Little things can make a big difference when you're tired or feeling overwhelmed.

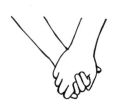

- ◆ Get up and move! Exercise is important for your partner. Offer to join them for a walk, workout, or swim. Urge them to try a prenatal yoga class with a friend.

- ◆ Think of things you can do around the home that are risky during pregnancy. Things like handling raw meat, changing cat litter, or scooping dog poop are all good ways to help. Some tasks may be risky or harder as your partner's body changes, like lifting heavy things or doing things that need a ladder. Make a list of your ideas and show it to your partner. What do they want to add or change?

- ◆ Have safe sex. STIs can harm an unborn baby. Some can even cause miscarriage. If you have an STI, tell your partner and their provider.

- ◆ Stay healthy. It's not helpful for anyone to get sick. Wash your hands often and get your own vaccines. Stay away from people who are sick or wear a mask around them. If you are sick, do your best not to share your germs with your partner.

- ◆ Make a plan to change your unhealthy habits. See chapter 17 to learn more.

Unhealthy Habits	Yes	Sometimes	No
I drink beer, wine, hard seltzer, or liquor			
I smoke or chew tobacco			
I vape or use e-cigarettes			
I use illegal drugs or prescription drugs not from my doctor			
I have unprotected sex or have many partners			
I use marijuana or cannabis products			

Chapter 4

What You Eat, Drink, and Breathe

Almost everything you take into your body can affect your baby's growth and health. Many things you eat, drink, and breathe pass into your baby's blood. Being good to your body is important for both of you.

Some kinds of foods, drinks, and drugs can harm your growing fetus. You are the only one who can make sure your baby is not exposed to these things. It can be hard to change habits, but it can make a big difference to your baby.

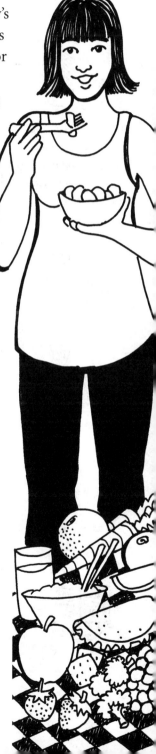

Look in this chapter for:

Healthy eating for you and baby

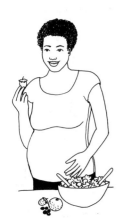

Eating well is one of the most important things you can do right now. Healthy foods help your body stay strong and your baby's brain and body grow.

Choosing healthy foods is a habit that gets easier the more you do it. Start small by finding healthier options for a few foods each time you shop. Whole grain breads are better than white. Fresh fruit and veggies are often better than canned. Yogurt can be just as tasty as ice cream. Veggies can go into a smoothie if you don't like eating them on a plate!

"When I shop for food, I try to get many kinds of food in my cart. Then my meals aren't boring."

What should I eat?

Your body will feel the best if you eat a variety of foods. Choose a few different things from each food group each day.

The five food groups

Vegetables

Broccoli, squash, yam, carrots, kale, spinach, collards, bok choy—dark green or bright colored veggies are best. You can eat fresh, frozen, canned, or dried, or drink 100 percent vegetable juice.

Fruits

Oranges, papaya, apples, melons, berries, prunes, raisins – bright colored fruits are best. You can eat fresh, frozen, canned, or dried, or drink 100 percent fruit juice.

Grains

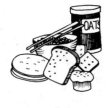

Bread, cereal, crackers, pasta, oatmeal, tortillas, and pita are made from grains. Look for "whole grain" on the label. Oats, quinoa, brown rice, buckwheat, whole corn flour, and wheat berries are all whole grains.

Protein foods

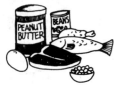

Fish, chicken, turkey, lean meat, and eggs are good animal sources* of protein. Beans, peas, nuts, seeds, and tofu are good vegan sources of protein. Many meat alternatives (seitan, TVP,

*Some meats and fish should be avoided. Keep reading to learn more.

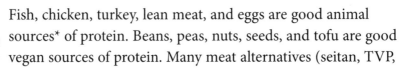

veggie burgers, and other plant-based meats) are high in protein, but some are very high in sodium. Check labels and talk to your provider about what options are best for you.

Calcium-rich foods – Dairy and non-dairy

Pasteurized milk, yogurt, hard cheeses, cottage cheese, and ice cream are good dairy sources of calcium. Sardines, anchovies, spinach, collards, rhubarb, beans, sesame seeds, soy nuts, chia seeds, eggs, and blackstrap molasses are good non-dairy sources. Look for "calcium added" on soy or nut milks, orange juice, cereals, tofu, egg replacers, and bread. You can also take a calcium supplement*.

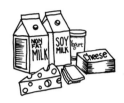

*Supplement: An extra amount of a nutrient (like a vitamin).

On the side – Fats

Oils and fats are part of healthy eating, especially while pregnant. Oils from plants are the best choices—olive oil, nut oil, grapeseed oil. Avocados, nuts, olives, and some fish also have a lot of healthy fats. Many healthy fats have omega-3 fatty acids, which are good for you and baby.

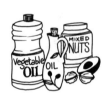

Water and healthy drinks

Most people don't drink enough water. It's very important to drink at least 8 to 12 cups of water each day. It can be hot or cold, plain or flavored with slices of fruit or fresh ginger. Keep a bottle of water with you everywhere you go. Not getting enough water can cause problems for you and for baby.

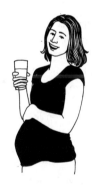

Water is best, but having some other healthy drinks is okay, too. Milk or 100 percent fruit or vegatable juice are good choices. Broths and soup also count. A little bit of coffee or tea can be fine, too. Avoid too much caffeine, sodium, or sugar. Energy drinks and soda are not good for you or baby.

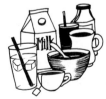

How much should I eat?

How much food you should eat is different for each person. It depends on how old, tall, heavy, and active you are. Some health issues can also change how much and what kind of food is best for you and baby. Talk to your provider about your nutritional needs while pregnant.

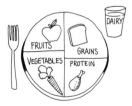

Make sure fruits and veggies fill half your dinner plate.

"I went to www.MyPlate.gov to find my own prenatal nutrition needs and showed it to my midwife. They helped me find ways to make it work for me!"

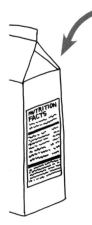

*Nutrients:
Vitamins, minerals, and other things in food that people need to be healthy.

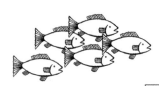

"I really miss my sushi and poke, but better safe than sorry."

For most people, it is best to fill half your plate with fruits and veggies, and the rest with a mix from the dairy, grain, and protein groups.

Learn to read food labels

Packaged foods all have nutrient* fact labels. Check the label to find how big a serving is, so you know how much to eat. This label will also show you how much of each nutrient is in each serving. This is a great way to check for sodium or sugar.

What shouldn't I eat?

Some foods are not safe during pregnancy. Others are only safe in small amounts.

Do not have:

- ◆ raw fish or shellfish or cold uncooked seafood.
- ◆ any kind of undercooked meat. Use a meat thermometer while cooking.
- ◆ cold hot dogs or lunch meat. Always heat until steaming.
- ◆ raw or runny eggs. Cook until whites and yolks are firm.
- ◆ raw or unpasteurized dairy products or juice.
- ◆ liver. It can have toxic levels of vitamin A and copper.
- ◆ alcohol. See pages 50 and 51 to learn more.

A note on fish

Some fish is very good for you. Choose 8 to 12 ounces of salmon, cod, anchovies, tilapia, sardines, shrimp, pollock, "fish sticks," catfish, or light canned tuna each week.

Other fish have a lot of mercury in them. Mercury is toxic to unborn babies and young kids. Avoid high-mercury fish like shark, swordfish, king mackerel, tilefish, bigeye tuna, and orange roughy. Certain rivers, lakes, and parts of the ocean can also be unsafe to eat fish from. Check with the local health department before eating fish caught by family or friends.

Limit how much you have of these:

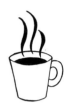

- ◆ Caffeine—Less than 200 mg a day. That could be a small cup of coffee, a cup of black tea, or a small soda pop or dark chocolate bar. Ask the pharmacy before taking medicine for colds or headaches. Check the labels on sports drinks. Avoid drinks, herbs, or pills that say they give you energy or improve focus.

- ◆ Vitamin A—No more than 5,000 IU. Vitamin A (retinol) is good, but too much can be toxic for you and baby. You'll get all you need from taking a prenatal vitamin and eating meats, eggs, and colorful fruits and veggies. Don't take extra vitamin A or eat liver.

- ◆ Salt—Ask your provider. A little salt (sodium) is good and can provide iodine. But too much can raise blood pressure, which is not good while pregnant.

- ◆ Sugar and sweeteners—Ask your provider. Pregnancy can change how your body handles sugar. Check labels for "added sugars" or sweeteners.

- ◆ Extra vitamins, herbs, or other supplements. Keep reading to learn more.

Going out to eat

It can be helpful to get food while you're out or treat yourself to take-out. But, beware! Many restaurant foods are high in salt, fat, and sugar. Restaurants also often serve very large meals. By making smart choices when you order out, you can stay healthy while you enjoy treating yourself.

- ◆ Choose meat or sides that are baked or grilled, not fried.

- ◆ Get dressings or sauces "on the side" and use just a bit.

- ◆ Have salad, slaw, or veggies instead of fries or chips.

- ◆ Drink water or milk instead of soda pop.

- ◆ Ask for a to-go box when you order, so you can save half for tomorrow.

"I love having leftovers. I write the date on a piece of tape and put it on the container. Then it's easy to throw out food if I keep it too long."

What else you and baby need

Eating healthy is very important. But, it's very hard to get enough of all the vitamins and minerals you need in pregnancy just from food. Prenatal vitamins are full of the right nutrients to keep you and your baby healthy and strong. Look at the label to see exactly what is in each kind. Look for "100% DV" (daily value) so you don't have to take any extra supplements. Too much of a good thing can be very bad.

Prenatal vitamins

If you are a tween or teen, you are still growing! You need enough nutrients for both you and baby to keep growing.

Choose a prenatal vitamin that has everything you need. Two of the most important ingredients to look for are folic acid and iron.

Folic acid (folate) is one of the most important things in a prenatal vitamin. Folate helps prevent birth defects in the brain and spinal cord. If you are not pregnant yet, it's best to start taking it at least three months before getting pregnant.

"My doctor said it was the iron in my vitamins that was making it hard to poop. Now I eat more fiber and drink more water and it's no problem!"

Iron is another very important thing to look for. Iron helps your body make enough blood for both you and baby. It also helps prevent anemia (too few red blood cells). Iron is in most prenatal vitamins because it's hard to get enough from food.

Once you find a vitamin with enough folic acid and iron, look at what else they have in them. **Iodine** is needed for baby's brain and bone growth, before and after birth. **DHA** (omega-3 fatty acid) helps baby's brain grow. **Calcium** and **vitamin D** are good for baby's bones. Look for other good things like **vitamin C**, **vitamin A**, **vitamin E**, **B vitamins**, and **zinc**.

Bring the prenatal vitamin you've chosen to your next checkup. Also bring any other supplements or teas you might be taking. Your provider can help make sure you're getting what you and baby need, but not too much.

"My burps smelled so much like vitamins all morning. Now I take them at bed time so I can sleep through it!"

Prenatal vitamins come in large pills, small capsules, liquid, powder drink mix, and even gummies. Find one that has what you need and is easy for you to take. If it upsets your stomach or is hard to remember in the morning, try taking it at night. It's important to take it each day.

Learn about WIC

The **Women, Infants, and Children Program (WIC)** is a nutrition program for those who are pregnant, gave birth recently, or are breastfeeding. It also serves babies and young kids.

WIC is found in many public health clinics, hospitals, schools, and housing centers. Once you are signed up, you can get checks to buy healthy foods. You can also learn about prenatal care, get help with breastfeeding, and learn about caring for baby. WIC staff can also help connect you with other resources near you.

If your provider doesn't know how to contact your local WIC office, see chapter 17 for WIC's website and phone numbers.

What if I have an eating disorder?

You and baby both need enough nutrients right now. See page 93 for tips on how to handle eating while pregnant.

What if I have a special diet?

Some people do not eat certain foods due to allergies, health problems, or their beliefs. It is important to tell your provider if you have a special diet. They can help you make sure to get enough nutrients using foods you do eat and extra supplements.

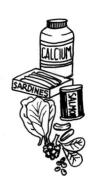

If you don't eat meat, you need to make sure you get enough protein, iron, and vitamins B12, and D.

If you don't eat dairy or eggs, you'll also need to get enough calcium.

Look back at page 42 for ideas for healthy foods.

What if I can't afford organic foods?

A "USDA Organic" label means the farmer followed the rules on how that food was grown and processed. Organic foods may have a bit more of the good stuff (nutrients and omega-3s) and less of the bad stuff (toxins and pesticides). Organic farming is good for the Earth, but it may not make a big difference to your health.

The downside of organic foods is that they are more expensive. And they don't stay fresh as long. Plus, just because a food is

"I buy organic when it's on sale. But I always wash or rinse any produce, no matter what the label says."

organic, doesn't mean it's healthy. Check labels for salt, sugar, and fat.

What's most important is to get lots of fresh, healthy foods each day. Keep these tips in mind:

- Buy fruits and veggies that are in season.
- Buy food grown nearby when you can. (You can use WIC or food stamps at farmer's markets.)
- Wash fresh fruits and veggies before cutting, cooking, or eating. Scrubbing or using mild soap can get off extra dirt, wax, or chemicals.
- Throw away the outside layers of foods like cabbage or onion.
- Rinse rice and other grains before cooking.

Eating things that aren't food

Some pregnant people crave things that are not food. Some things, like ice, are not harmful. But others can be dangerous or even toxic, like dirt, soap, ashes, sand, paint, or burnt matches. This is called **pica** and it is often a sign that your body isn't getting enough nutrients. Tell your provider right away if you start wanting to eat anything that is not really food.

Food safety – Germs

People often get sick from food that isn't clean or is not cooked enough. Food that is not fresh or that is not stored well can also go bad quickly. Food poisoning is dangerous while pregnant. Make sure you handle, cook, and store food safely, at home and on the go.

Listeria

Listeria bacteria are often found in unclean food or drink, or foods that are not cooked enough. Listeria infection, called **listeriosis**, can make anyone very sick. It is very dangerous in pregnancy and can cause miscarriage, stillbirth, or preterm birth. Infected babies may be born very small or very ill.

How can I protect myself and baby?

Follow these food safety tips to avoid listeriosis and other food-borne illnesses:

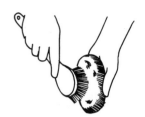

- Wash fruits and veggies before cutting, cooking, or eating them.
- Cook all meats, poultry, and fish well. Canned fish is okay cold.
- Avoid raw fish, like sushi, and other raw meats.
- Avoid raw sprouts.
- Heat prepared meats (hot dogs, lunch meat) until steaming before eating.
- Avoid soft cheeses like feta or queso fresco, or cheese with blue veins. Other cheeses like cheddar or mozzarella, cream cheese, and cottage cheese are safer.
- Do not drink raw milk, raw yogurt, or cheese made from raw milk..
- Wash your hands after using the bathroom, helping a child wipe, or changing a diaper.

Keep things clean

- Wash your hands with soap and water before and after touching uncooked food.
- Cut raw meat on its own cutting board. Wash it well after each use.
- Rinse or wash fruits and vegetables before cutting or eating them.
- Use soap or disinfectant to clean the counters after cutting raw meat.

Keep things fresh

- Set your refrigerator to 37°F (2.8°C).
- Eat fresh prepared foods, such as roast chicken, salads, pizza, or sandwiches soon after buying them.
- Store leftovers in a sealed container in the refrigerator within a few hours of cooking and eat them within a few days.

Heat things up

- ◆ Cook all meats, poultry, fish, and eggs well. Use a meat thermometer if you're not sure.
- ◆ Keep foods hot until you are ready to serve them.

What you do with your body matters

Most of us have at least a few bad habits. Some may not be a big deal, but others can put both you and baby at serious risk. Making healthy choices gets easier the more we do it.

Some things are dangerous for baby

Anything you put into your body can also go into baby's body. Drugs, cigarettes, nicotine*, and alcohol are very dangerous for baby. They can cause lifelong problems for baby and even lead to premature birth, miscarriage, or stillbirth. There are many ways to get help quitting these habits. Be honest with your provider if you are smoking or using drugs. They may be able to find ways to help you quit.

*Nicotine: A chemical in tobacco that is very harmful.

Medicines

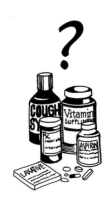

Most medicines you take can be passed from your body to your baby's. It's important to make sure none of them are harmful. Make a list of everything you take daily or as needed and show it to your provider. This should include:

- ◆ medicines you were prescribed before you were pregnant.
- ◆ drugs you can buy at the store, like aspirin, ibuprofen, laxatives, or allergy medicine.
- ◆ vitamins, supplements, herbs, or special drinks.

If your provider or pharmacy tells you that any of them are unsafe for baby, ask if there is a safer option for you to take.

"My anxiety medicine wasn't safe while pregnant, but my doctor found a safer option for me."

Alcohol

Alcohol can harm a child for life. When you drink, the alcohol goes from your blood stream right into baby's. Alcohol can hurt an unborn baby's growing brain. They could have disabilities that last their whole life. These are called fetal alcohol spectrum disorders (FASDs)*. Alcohol can also cause baby to be born too soon, be very small, or be stillborn.

Is there a safe kind of alcohol? How much is too much?

The harm alcohol can cause to baby is serious and can't be undone. *There is no known safe amount to drink while pregnant.* There is no safe kind of alcohol, even if it doesn't taste strong or you only have a little.

Those first weeks of pregnancy are very important to baby's brain development. Any amount of alcohol can cause damage. Stop drinking as soon as you think you could be pregnant. The safest thing is not to drink at all.

Is it hard to stop drinking?

You don't have to be an alcoholic for your unborn baby to be harmed by what you drink. Many people drink out of habit or because the people around them are drinking. Switching to a non-alcoholic drink may be all you need to do.

Ask for help

- ◆ Talk to your provider about how they can help you quit. They may know of a support group or a program that can help.
- ◆ Visit **FindTreatment.gov** to learn more about how to get treatment and what to expect. You can also call **1-800-662-HELP (4357)**.
- ◆ Tell your partner and friends that you want to quit. Quitting may be hard but will be the best thing for you and for baby.

See page 294 for more resources.

Cigarettes

Your baby needs the oxygen you breathe in the air. That oxygen passes into their body through your blood. But, so do any toxins and chemicals you breathe in. Cigarette smoke contains thousands of chemicals. Nearly a hundred of those cause cancer and many more are toxic (poisonous). Smoking puts you at risk

***Fetal alcohol spectrum disorders:** FASDs can cause a child to grow more slowly and look different from other kids. They can cause problems with how a child thinks, learns, eats, sleeps, or behaves.

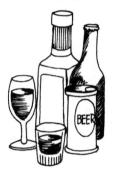

of cancer, heart disease, stroke, lung disease, and other severe health and dental problems.

If you smoke while you are pregnant, all of these toxins are passed to baby, too.

When you smoke:

◆ baby's heart beats very fast.

◆ baby does not get enough oxygen, which can cause brain damage.

◆ baby is likely to be born too soon (premature) or very small (low birth weight).

◆ you are more at risk for a miscarriage or stillbirth.

◆ you are more at risk for dangerous problems during pregnancy and birth.

"I learned that menthol cigarettes have stuff in them that is really bad for you and make it even harder to quit!"

After birth, babies of smokers may have more colds, breathing problems, and ear infections than other kids.

Some kinds of cigarettes, cigars, and smoking tobacco have even more toxins in them that can harm both you and baby.

Secondhand smoke (smoke from other people)

You do not have to be a smoker to be harmed by cigarette smoke. Any smoke in the air around you can get into your lungs and your bloodstream. This is called secondhand smoke. Secondhand smoke has the same toxins and can cause most of the same damage that smoking can.

"When I asked my sister not to smoke around me, she decided to quit smoking! She said doing it for baby was the perfect reason."

When you are pregnant, the things that go into your body go into baby's, too. Secondhand smoke from someone else can affect baby and you as much as if you were smoking yourself.

Try to stay away from people who are smoking. Ask your friends and family who smoke not to do it while you are with them, even outside or in the car with a window down. Don't spend time in smoky places.

E-cigarettes (vaping)

NO!

Vaping is very popular, but it is not good for you. The vapor you breathe in has most of the same toxic chemicals in it as cigarette smoke. Some kinds of vape liquid ("e-juice") have other drugs in them or oils that can make you very sick.

E-cigarette vapor can harm baby's heart and brain development. It can cause baby to be born too early or too small. It can also cause miscarriage or stillbirth.

Smokeless tobacco

Tobacco products that you chew, suck, or sniff still have nicotine and other harmful chemicals. These toxins pass through the skin in your mouth or are swallowed with your spit. Once in your bloodstream, they go right into baby's bloodstream. This puts baby at risk of birth defects and damage to the brain and lungs. It can cause baby to be born too early or too small. It can also cause miscarriage or stillbirth.

How to quit smoking*

The best time to quit using tobacco is *before* you get pregnant. If you can't do that, the next best time is as soon as you can! Quitting by the 15th week of your pregnancy gives your baby the best shot at being healthy. But it's never too late to quit! Any time you quit smoking is that much better for you and for baby.

*We use the word "smoking" a lot, but this includes any kinds of tobacco use. Chew, snuff, strips, and gels are all harmful in pregnancy.

Ask for help

Talk to your provider about how they can help you quit. They may know of a support group or a program that can help.

Visit *SmokeFree.gov* to learn more about making a Quit Plan, helpful apps, and signing up for texts. You can also chat or talk to an expert. You can also call **1-800-QUIT-NOW (1-800-784-8669)**.

See Page 294 for more resources.

Make a quit plan

People start smoking for many reasons, then it becomes a habit. Over time, you start to crave it at certain times and in certain situations. The longer you have smoked, the harder it can be to stop. Making a plan for when to quit, how to cope with cravings, and what to do when it feels hard can help you stick with it.

Here are some things to think about:

Why do I want to stop? (for baby's health, $$$, or...)

_____

_____

Do the math. See how much smoking costs you!

How much $$$ will I save?

- How much could I save every week by not buying cigarettes?

_____
packs per day   ×   7   =   _____
packs per week

_____ $_____ $_____
packs per week   ×   **cost of each pack**   =   **cost per week**

What things make me want to smoke? (being around smokers, my lunch break, stress, or . . .)

_____
_____
_____
_____

Most cravings don't last long. Find something else to do for 10 minutes or so.

- four-song dance party
- Walk the dog around the block
- Go up and down the stairs
- Drink a tall glass of water
- Take 10 slow, deep breaths

What will I do when I want to smoke? (go for a walk, call a friend, chew gum, or . . .)

_____
_____
_____
_____

When will I quit? (Choose a date and time.)

_____

How will I quit? (Break all cigarettes, throw away ash trays, use the QuitGuide app, or . . .

_____
_____
_____
_____

Who can help? (My doctor, my partner, my friends, SmokeFree.gov, or . . .)

_____
_____
_____
_____

The day you quit

Get rid of all cigarettes and ashtrays in your home, car, and at work. Tell all your friends you have quit and ask for their help.

What will it be like? Quitting smoking feels different for everyone. The most common side effects are:

- feeling cranky or mad.
- having a hard time focusing.
- feeling sad or run down.
- having trouble sleeping.

The best distraction is to get your body moving. Take good care of yourself by taking a long walk or going out with non-smoking friends. Find fun and healthy ways to distract yourself when you want to smoke. Try a new recipe, go see a movie, try a new craft hobby, or do a video call with someone you haven't seen in a while.

Most people have less cravings after two or three weeks. Just take it one day at a time!

Celebrate!

Breaking bad habits is hard work. Reward yourself! Every day you make it without smoking, do something to celebrate. Make a smoothie, get your nails done, take a prenatal yoga class . . . whatever feels like a treat!

Staying smoke-free

Being smoke-free is the safest and healthiest for both you and those around you. Babies and young kids who breathe smoke have more colds and ear infections. They are at high risk of breathing problems and lung infections. Babies who are around smoke may not grow well and are at higher risk of SIDS*.

The best way to stay smoke-free is to not cheat at all. Even one puff from a cigarette can make your body start craving it all over again. If you do give in and smoke, don't give up! It's a hard process. Just start again, one day at a time.

***SIDS:** Sudden Infant Death Syndrome is when a baby dies in their sleep area with no known cause of death. See chapter 14 for more on SIDS and sleep safety.

Drug use

Any drugs can be very dangerous for a pregnant person and their unborn baby. Many drugs pass through the umbilical cord and into baby's body. This puts you at high risk of miscarriage or stillbirth. It puts baby at risk of severe birth defects or being born too soon or very small. These problems can last for baby's whole life.

Marijuana (pot)

Using marijuana during pregnancy is not recommended. There is not enough evidence to know what kind or how much is safe for baby. Some studies show that it may put baby at risk of problems with their brain or behavior throughout their life.

A lot of people don't think of marijuana as a serious drug. It's legal in many states and can be smoked, vaped, dabbed, eaten, swallowed, or spread on the skin. Some cannabis (marijuana) products have a chemical called THC* that causes changes in how your mind and body feel (a "high"). People use this type of marijuana to feel good, relax, or cope with certain health problems. Some CBD** products have almost no THC, so they may interact with your brain in certain ways, but do not cause a high. People often use this type of marijuana to help with anxiety, attention span, or pain.

Any type of marijuana use during pregnancy can put you and your baby at risk. If you use pot or CBD products for health reasons, talk to your provider. There may be a safer option for you to feel good without the risk.

*THC: The substance in marijuana that affects how your brain processes pleasure, memory, and thought. It causes the "high".

**CBD: Cannabidiol is the substance in marijuana that may affect some parts of your brain, but does not cause a high.

Prescription drugs

Many people who take drugs think it's safe if it is something they could get from a doctor. But, drugs like sleeping pills, cough syrup, and pain medicine are easy to get hooked on. Some people take more than they're supposed to or use them with alcohol or other drugs. These are very harmful to your body, even when you are not pregnant. When you are, they are very harmful to both you and baby.

Any of these drugs can harm your baby. If you use this way, it's important to quit. Be sure to tell your provider all the drugs you take, how much and how often. They can help you find safer options to help with your problems, and connect you to better help.

Other illegal drugs (street drugs)

Strong drugs, like cocaine, heroin, meth, PCP, or xylazine are extremely dangerous for unborn babies. When you get high, so does your baby. Even if it makes you feel good for a short time, it can cause lifelong harm to your child.

Drugs can cause:

◆ miscarriage or stillbirth.

◆ preterm birth or low birthweight*, which can cause serious problems.

◆ a baby born addicted to drugs who will deal with painful withdrawal after birth.

◆ a child who has trouble with their health, learning, or behavior their whole life.

*__Low birthweight__: A baby who has not grown well before birth. They are very small and often have many serious health problems.

Using drugs even a few times can cause serious harm to an unborn baby. If you have a drug habit, now is the time to get help and quit. Quitting may not be fast or easy, but you and your baby are worth it. The sooner you stop drinking, smoking, or using drugs, the better for both of you. It's hard, but you can do it!

Fentanyl—Most risky of all

One of the most dangerous drugs right now is *illegally made fentanyl* (IMF). **Fentanyl** is a very strong opioid* that is used in health care for severe pain control. It is so strong, that drug dealers make it illegally to get more people addicted so they'll buy more drugs. This fentanyl is 50 times stronger than heroin and can kill you in just one use. It has no smell or taste and can be a in a liquid, powder, or pill form. It is added to other street drugs, like heroin, cocaine, meth, or xylazine (*tranq*). It is also made to look like popular prescription drugs, like oxycodone (Percocet). It is also sold on the street as eye drops, nose spray, or even candy.

*__Opioid:__ A type of drug used to reduce pain. Often known as **pain killers**, they are very addictive. Opioid overdose causes tens of thousands of deaths each year.

Save a life!

Naloxone can save someone from an opioid overdose. Even a small amount of fentanyl can kill very quickly.

If you *think* someone is overdosing:

◆ Call 9-1-1
◆ Give naloxone
◆ Try to keep them awake
◆ Lay them on their side
◆ Stay there until help arrives

Naloxone is easy to get, carry, and use. Learn how to spot and respond to an overdose, and where to get free naloxone near you at *naloxoneforall.org*

See page 294 for tools to help you quit. You can also visit *FindTreatment.gov* or call **1-800-662-HELP (4357)**.

Quitting drinking, smoking, or using drugs

A few ideas to make quitting a bad habit easier:

- ◆ Stay away from others who are doing it.
- ◆ Spend time with people who don't drink, smoke, or do drugs.
- ◆ Get active. Fresh air and exercise help your body focus on feeling good.
- ◆ Do something else when you feel like using. Go to a movie or call a friend.
- ◆ Get support. Tell your loved ones you are quitting and want their help. Join a support group for people trying to quit.

Don't give up! You and baby are worth it.

If people around you are using

Keeping yourself and baby safe is one of your biggest jobs right now. Driving after you have been drinking or using drugs is very dangerous. So is riding with a driver who has been drinking or using, even if they seem okay.

If your driver has been drinking or using drugs you can:

- ◆ drive yourself.
- ◆ take a cab home.
- ◆ ask someone who has not been drinking or using for a ride.
- ◆ stay with friends.

Tips for partners

- Fill up your partner's water bottle when it's empty. Bring water and snacks for your partner when you go out together.

- Make time to take walks with your partner, and to relax together. It's important for them to be active each day but to also get extra rest.

- Clear the air. Baby breathes what your partner breathes. Don't let anyone smoke or vape around them, even outside or in the car. Take over jobs that have fumes, like using strong cleaners or putting gas in the car.

- Stop bad habits. Your drinking, smoking, and using drugs puts your partner and baby at risk. It will also be much harder for them to quit if you are using. Get all drugs and alcohol out of the house. Don't use around your partner. Now is the time to get help and get clean.

Chapter 5

Health Care for You and Baby

It's important to have a prenatal health checkup at least once a month. Even if you're feeling great, these checkups are one key to staying healthy. These visits to your health care provider help find and treat problems early. Some problems you may not even know you have. Checkups also give you time to ask questions.

You may be able to use the doctor you already go to. If not, you will need to choose a prenatal care provider and a place to give birth. Your choices depend on what kind of care you want before and during birth. The health insurance you have may limit your choices. This chapter will help you get started.

Words about your care

Some words you may hear are maternity care, prenatal care, and obstetrical care. They all mean the care you get for your pregnancy. We will use the words "prenatal care."

Words for visits to your provider include appointments, visits, and checkups. We will use "visits" and "checkups."

Some words used for the birth of a baby are birth, childbirth, or labor and delivery. Usually we will use "birth." Your care *after* birth is usually called **postpartum care**.

Choices in prenatal care and birth

The place you give birth, the kind of care you want, and the provider go together. These are very personal choices, so take some time to decide. You want to be comfortable with your provider.

Know what your insurance pays for

Start by talking to your insurance company, employee benefits office, or health clinic. Find out:

- what kinds of prenatal and birth care does your plan pay for?
- how much will you have to pay yourself?
- what options do you have?

The answers to these questions will help you know how much choice you have for place and provider.

If you don't have health insurance now, call or visit your local public health clinic. You may be able to sign up for Medicaid. There also are community health centers that offer low-cost care.

Learn enough to make a good choice

To make these choices, it helps to know what happens during birth. Reading chapters 6 and 10 will give you a good start. (Use the Glossary in chapter 17 to find the meanings of words you don't know.)

If you think you want to change providers, you can. But it's easier not to have to change.

Some people choose their doctor or midwife first. Whoever you choose will work at a specific medical center or clinic. They will have preferences for the types of delivery they do.

Other people feel strongly about where and how they give birth. They want to choose a birth place first and then find a provider who delivers there.

If you're not sure where to go for care, call:

◆ your insurance plan.

◆ local public health office.

◆ community clinic.

◆ nearby hospital.

Choosing a place to give birth

Different kinds of birth places are good for different reasons. (Read more on the next pages.)

◆ **Hospital**—all services in one place, may have a focus on using medical ways of birth.

◆ **Birth center in a hospital**—a blend of medical and natural ways of birth, more choices between medical and natural ways of birth.

◆ **Birth center outside a hospital**—more personal care, easier to use natural ways of birth, for people with problem-free pregnancies.

◆ **Your home**—most personal and family-centered, easiest to use natural ways of birth, for people with problem-free pregnancies.

There are a lot of things to think about before choosing where to have your baby. What kind of birth do you want to have?

Ask your friends where they gave birth and what kinds of medical things were done. Ask what they liked or disliked about the provider and place. Did they use any drugs? Could they get up and move when they wanted?

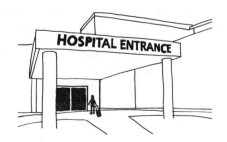

Hospitals and birth centers in hospitals

Hospitals offer all birth services in one place. But not all hospitals have birth care. Look for one with a birth center. A birth center has private rooms set up just for having babies. It looks and feels less like a hospital. Medical machines are covered up and lights are dim. It's quieter than a regular maternity floor.

Things to think about before choosing birth in a hospital:

- You may have many different nurses and doctors or midwives during labor and birth.

- If you want medicine for pain or to help you rest, you can have it.

- If there is trouble during the birth or you need surgery (cesarean section*), it can be done right there.

*Cesarean section: Surgical birth of a baby. See chapter 10, page 169, to learn more.

- You and baby will stay there one to two days, maybe longer. Nurses will be there to help you recover and teach you how to care for baby. There will be people to help with breastfeeding.

- There are staff to help you with insurance, social services, birth certificates, and other big decisions.

In some hospitals, providers and nurses have a set way of doing things. So, they may expect you to come in, give birth, and recover a certain way. These ways could be simple things like having you wear a hospital gown and lying in bed during labor. Or, they may want to use medical tools early in labor, before trying other things. In the hospital, the use of pain medicine, vaginal exams, and fetal monitors is more likely. A **hospital birth center** may be more open to letting things happen on their own.

"I had a birth plan at the hospital, but I was glad my partner was there to keep reminding them about my goals, even when I got really tired."

If you want to give birth in a hospital, think about how you want it to be. If you feel strongly about not rushing labor, make a plan with your provider. See chapter 9 about making a birth plan.

Private birth centers and birth at home

You may want a more natural birth. You may want to avoid medicines and monitors. You may want to wear your own clothes and move around during labor. You are more likely to be able to have this kind of birth outside of the hospital.

A birth center or home birth is safest for those who have low-risk pregnancies. You are at "low risk" for problems if you:

- are under 35 years of age,
- are expecting only one baby, and
- have no existing health problems like diabetes.

Of course, sometimes problems start during pregnancy. Your provider may believe a hospital birth is best. It is important to be able to get the care you and baby need if there are problems.

Birth center

A private birth center is like a hospital birth center without the hospital. The rooms are set up like bedrooms. Some may have a kitchen, bathroom, or hot tub, too. Most births are done with midwives. Some doctors deliver at birth centers, too. You go to the birth center when you're in labor, and often leave just a few hours after birth.

Planned home birth

You may want to have your baby at home. This is most often done with a midwife, sometimes with a doctor. You purchase the supplies and your provider comes to you when you're in labor. Basic care after birth is done at home, too.

You may feel most comfortable and private at home. Your kids may be able to be at the birth, too.

Things to know before choosing birth outside a hospital

- Most births do not have problems. Most people do not need drugs or medical help. It helps to have providers who know natural ways to help with birth. But in many areas there are very few doctors or midwives who will deliver in a birth center or at home.

- You will have more choices in labor and birth at home or a birth center. You also will get more help using natural ways to cope with pain.

- Pain medicines (narcotics and epidurals) **cannot** be used there. If you end up needing them, you must go to the hospital.

- When problems happen, they can happen fast. It's important for your midwife to have a trusted doctor to call if there are problems. It could be for advice or to send you to the hospital for care.

- Birth centers often have you go home just a few hours after the baby is born. After a home birth, you won't have to go anywhere.

- Make sure the midwife has a doctor to call in case of problems.

- Think ahead. You and your partner probably will both be exhausted. At home there will be no nurse, midwife, or doctor nearby. You may need care yourself. Starting to breastfeed and care for your newborn may give you lots of questions.

- Be sure you know an expert to call if you need help. Also, have an experienced family member or friend, or a doula, to care for and encourage you.

- Though the cost of a birth center is far less than a hospital birth, it is not always covered by insurance.

In the unlikely case of an emergency, think about:

- What hospital would your midwife send you to? How far away is it? To be safe, you should be able to get there in less than 20 minutes.

- If you need to move to a hospital, it can be hard. You would likely have to call 9-1-1 and ride in an ambulance.

Choosing your health care provider

Every pregnant person needs a prenatal provider who is well trained and has delivered lots of babies. You also want someone you trust to give you the best care. This person will be very important to you for the next seven or eight months. Get a list of providers from your health plan.

These are the kinds of health care providers who give prenatal and birth care:

Obstetrician (OB): A medical doctor (MD) or osteopathic doctor (DO) with special training in pregnancy and childbirth. An OB (also called an "OB-GYN") can do cesarean surgery.

Midwife: A certified nurse midwife (CNM) is a nurse with special training to deliver babies. A certified professional midwife (CPM) or licensed midwife (LM) is trained as a midwife and is not also a nurse. Use only a midwife who is certified or licensed.

Some are also naturopathic doctors (ND) who provide prenatal care at their office. Many midwives do births in hospitals and in birth centers. Some do home births. None do cesareans.

Family practice doctor: A medical doctor (MD) or osteopathic doctor (DO) who cares for people of all ages. Some family doctors deliver babies but many don't. They can care for your other medical needs and your baby after birth.

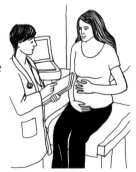

Note: In this book, we will use the word "midwife" for all kinds of professional midwives. We will use **doctor** to mean an OB, MD, or DO.

The best provider for you

Talk to a few providers before you choose. (This should be free.) One of the most important things is to choose someone you can talk openly with and feel safe. There may be things about your health or body that are uncomfortable to talk about but could affect your pregnancy. Find someone you can be honest with.

Reading chapters 5, 8, 9, and 10 will help you know what questions you have before you talk to them.

Things to know before choosing

If there is something you feel strongly about, ask about it now. You want a provider who is right for you. Ask these questions.

"I looked on the internet at sites that rate doctors. But I wasn't sure that the ratings were true. So I didn't really use them. I trusted my own gut feeling."

- *What training have you had in labor and delivery? Are you certified? How many babies have you delivered?*
- *Are there other doctors or midwives who help care for your patients? Will I get to meet them?*
- *Who can I call nights or weekends if I have a question or an emergency?*
- *Do you help people to deliver in the position (sitting, squatting, in tub) that they feel is best?*
- *How do you help people handle pain without drugs? If I need something for pain, what do you use most often?*

*Episiotomy: A cut made in the skin around the vagina to widen the opening. This can make it easier for the baby to be born.

- *Do you try to avoid episiotomies*?*
- *Do you like for people to have a birth partner during labor and birth? How do you feel about having a doula there?*
- *What do you usually do if baby's due date passes?*
- *Do you support breastfeeding right after birth?*

Ask about your own needs:

- If you have a disability or a long-term health condition, speak a different language, or have other special needs or differences, ask questions. Have they cared for others with the same needs? Is their office easy to access? Do they have good interpreters or TTY phone lines?
- If you are thinking about not keeping the baby or need to end your pregnancy, will they support you?

Trauma is when something very scary or painful happens to you.

- If you have been through trauma, no matter how long ago, do they know how to support you?

Questions about cesarean section surgery:

- *When do you recommend a c-section?*
- *What ways do you help avoid c-sections?*
- *Do you support vaginal birth after c-section?*

See the end of chapter 7 for more notes on what to talk about and ask your provider about at your first visit.

Making your choice

Pick a provider you like and are comfortable with. Make sure they respect what you think. Choose one who:

- is well trained and certified by the state.
- listens to and respects your birth choices.
- has an office that is easy to get to and hours that work for you.
- can answer your questions by phone or email.
- can speak your language or use a medical interpreter.
- has easy access if you have a disability or a TTY phone line if you are hard of hearing.

Prenatal visits – Keep it up!

After your first appointment, your other checkups will be much shorter. After your provider asks and answers any questions, they will:

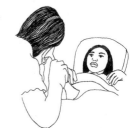

- check your blood pressure.
- see how much weight you've gained.
- measure your belly to see baby's growth.
- listen to baby's heartbeat.

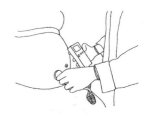

In the first 6 months of pregnancy, if all is going well, you will have a checkup about once a month. Starting at week 28, your provider will want to see you twice a month. Once you reach week 36, they will want you to have a checkup at least once a week until baby is born.

If you or baby have any problems or are high risk for health issues, you may need to go in more often. Ask your provider what to expect. You'll learn more about these checkups in chapters 7, 8, and 9. Each chapter has pages at the end to write down notes and questions.

Important things to talk about

A good provider knows that it takes more than just health care to live well. Your checkups are a good time to talk to your provider about any other worries or challenges you are having. They can help get you in touch with people and programs that can help.

- Paying for care – Do you need help getting health insurance for yourself or for baby? Do you know what care your plan covers?

- Safe housing – Do you have a safe place to live right now? And after baby is born?

- Transportation – Do you have a way to get to and from your checkups? Do you have a safe car seat for baby?

- Money – Raising a family costs money. Do you have a plan for how to make and save money? Do you know of resources in your area for pregnant and new families? It doesn't take a lot of money to be a wonderful parent. But it's a lot less stressful if you have enough money saved to pay for things.

- Labor support – Do you have someone to support you during labor? Ask about low cost or free doulas in your area.

- Child care – Do you have a plan for who will care for your baby while you work or go to school? You may be able to get help paying for childcare.

See page 284 for tips on how to find resources in your area.

Talking with your provider

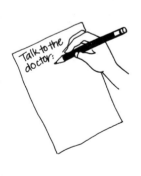

Your doctor or midwife will want to give you good care. But you must do your part, too. Your part is to be open and honest. Tell them how you feel and what worries you. Checkups are the best times to talk. But they will want you to call any time something serious comes up.

Write down concerns or questions as you think of them. This will help you remember what to ask at your next visit. There are places to write questions on the checkup pages in chapters 7, 8, and 9.

Any time you don't feel well

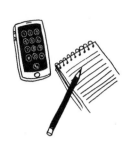

Be sure to call your doctor or midwife if you feel sick or have pain. See the list of warning signs in chapter 7.

Things to know before calling your provider (write in the answers here):

How do you feel different from usual?

_____

_____

How long have you been feeling this way?

_____

_____

How have the feelings changed?

_____

_____

Do you have a fever? (Take your temperature and write it down before you call.)

_____

Plan ahead – Care for baby

Your baby will need a lot of checkups, too. So you'll need to pick a provider before they are born. You won't have time after you have your baby.

Kinds of providers for babies and children:

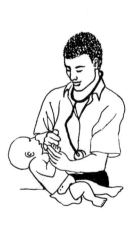

Pediatrician: A doctor (MD, DO, or ND) with special training in caring for babies and children

Pediatric nurse-practitioner: A nurse with special training in caring for babies and children

Family practice doctor: A doctor (MD, DO, or ND) who cares for people of all ages

If you already have a family doctor, that person could also care for your baby. If not, ask your doctor or midwife to suggest a doctor for baby. Check with your health plan to see which providers it covers. Ask your friends who their kids see and if they like them. It is best to meet with a few before picking one.

Some questions to ask:

- *Is the clinic or office easy to get to? (You will need to take your baby there often for checkups.) Do the office hours fit your schedule?*

- *Is the provider friendly and easy to talk to? Do they have time to answer questions? Do they have a nurse who can give advice by phone or email when you need it?*

- *Are they easy to reach in an emergency? Who can you call when they are away?*

- *Do their thoughts on baby care match yours? Think about how you feel about things like vaccines, breastfeeding, or sleep.*

Babies and children need to see their provider often even when they are not sick. These are called **well baby visits**. Most babies have about seven well-baby visits in their first year. See chapter 15 for more.

How will you pay for your baby's care?

If you have health insurance for your family, the plan will likely cover new babies. You must call the plan before birth to find out how to get your baby covered as they get older.

If you have no insurance for your baby, call your public health department or community clinic. These places can help you sign up for insurance or Medicaid for yourself and your baby. Ask about the Children's Health Insurance Program (CHIP).

Tips for partners

- Talk to your partner about what kind of birth they want. Read through what the options there are for where to give birth and how to choose.

- Help find out what is covered by insurance. (It could be their plan or yours.) Ask about having the baby added on.

- Go with your partner to meet providers. Talk together about who feels like the right fit.

- Talk with your partner about the kind of care you both want for baby. Go to meet providers and help your partner choose.

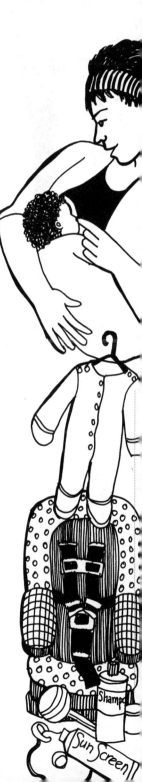

Chapter 6

Plan Ahead for Birth and Baby

Why is it important for you to think about birth and baby care now? It's best to know something about birth before you choose the kind of medical care you want. Also, it's never too early to start getting ready for your baby's birth. There is a lot to learn.

You'll have important decisions to make before you give birth. In the last months before birth, you will be busy and have less energy than now. You may need time to decide about birth options and breastfeeding. It can take time to get all the things you'll need for baby care. Once you have a baby, you will have very little time for shopping.

Look in this chapter for:

Preparing for Childbirth

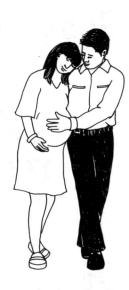

Learning about birth

Birthing a baby is a natural part of life. Having a delivery through your vagina (birth canal) is as normal as having sex. But that doesn't mean it's easy. The more prepared you are, the easier it is.

Most people feel proud and strong after they have a baby. They remember the excitement of birthing their baby more than the pain.

The best ways to get ready for birth:

- **Learn all about the stages of birth.** Learn the basics now by reading chapter 10. Read about different ways of giving birth. You may need to make some choices that aren't simple. Check out books and websites that you can trust. (See chapter 17 for resources.)

- **Choose a birth partner.** Having someone with you for support during birth will really help you. It might be your partner, a friend, or a relative. Think of a person who calms you down when you're upset. This person must really want to be in the room during the birth.

- **Take childbirth classes.** Sign up early. Taking a class is very important so you will know what to expect. Many hospitals, clinics, and childbirth groups give classes. Your birth partner should plan to go to these classes with you. Classes are most helpful if done early in your third trimester (30–36 weeks).

"I was really glad my partner stayed with me all the way through delivery. They were a huge help. It meant a lot that they were there to see what I was going through."

Start learning now

Bookmark chapter 10 of this book. It covers the basics of birth, stage by stage. It also tells about medical things (drugs, surgery) that might be done. Read about natural ways to cope with pain. Find out about epidurals and c-sections. Learn about what options and choices you may have.

Remember that every person and every birth is different. Also, many things have changed a lot over the years. Stories you've heard from older moms or grandmas don't have to be how things are for you.

How to cope with pain

Giving birth is not going to be comfortable. You can't avoid all the pain, even with pain medicine (drugs). The pain will be easier to cope with if you know what to expect. Knowing how to relax and having a birth partner also helps a lot. Keep in mind that the pain will go away between contractions and right after baby is born.

You may hear that it is easiest to have drugs for birth. Learn about the good and bad sides of drugs. Side effects and problems don't happen often, but they can be serious. Find out about the kinds of drugs available. Many people give birth with little or no pain medicine. Learn your options so you can choose what feels right to you.

Learn about cesarean section

A **cesarean section (c-section)** is major surgery to take a baby out of the uterus. You are given drugs in your spine so you can't feel much below the chest. The doctor makes a cut into your belly and then your uterus. Then baby is pulled out of the hole and you are stitched back up.

A c-section is necessary if there's an emergency with you or baby. Some problems can make a vaginal birth too risky. Then a c-section is the safest way to go.

See chapter 10 to learn more.

A cesarean section is surgery to get baby out fast.

Vaginal birth after cesarean

Many people who have a c-section end up having surgery for later babies, too. But, that's changing. Many parents want to have a vaginal birth next time. This is called vaginal birth after cesarean (VBAC, pronounced "vee-back"). VBAC is usually very safe, but can have some risk.

See chapter 10 to learn more.

Plan for support

Your birth team

Nurses and doctors will come and go during your labor. Even a midwife may not stay with you until it is time to push the baby out. It's good to have someone stay with you the whole time to help. This is your birth partner (sometimes called a labor coach).

Your birth partner can help you use the breathing and relaxation methods you learn in childbirth class. They can help you remember your goals and wishes, and help you to be as comfortable as possible.

Find someone who can go to classes with you. They may need to take time off from work or away from their family for the birth. You might ask two people, in case one can't be there the whole time.

Is your birth partner a good fit?

Giving birth is very personal. You want to be around people who will be calm, loving, and supportive. Try not to invite anyone who makes you stressed or uncomfortable. This can make labor harder.

Some people may be scared or upset by the idea of being part of a birth. Your partner or the baby's dad may not want to be there. If they feel that way, try to understand. Find someone else, maybe a good friend, your mom, or a doula.

How could a doula help you?

A birth doula is someone trained to help families in labor and birth and newborn care. A trained doula is there to support you by comforting, explaining, and encouraging. They can also support partners and guide them in how to help you. A doula can also help you understand what the provider says and explain what is going on.

People who have doulas often have shorter labors and better feelings about their births than those who give birth without doulas. There is less pain medicine use and fewer c-sections. They often have an easier time breastfeeding, and have healthier babies.

Most doulas work privately. Some hospitals have volunteer doulas for those who don't have one. Find out if there is a program in your area that offers doulas for little or no money to those in need. If you are an immigrant, you may find a doula who is from your culture and speaks your language. Ask your doctor or midwife to help you find one. (See chapter 17 for more.)

Arrange time off from work

You will need some time off from work after your baby is born (FMLA or maternity leave). Plan ahead.

Ask for as much maternity leave as you can get. It takes time to recover from birth. The first few months of parenthood can be very tiring. Also, you and your baby need time to get to know each other and bond with each other.

Learning about baby care

Learn all you can now. Most babies come home just one or two days after birth. You won't have time or energy for classes once baby's born. There's so much to know about, like breastfeeding, safe sleep, first aid and CPR* for babies, home safety, and car seat use.

*CPR: Cardio-pulmonary resuscitation. A way to save a life when a person isn't breathing. Infant CPR is very different from CPR for adults.

There are many ways to learn. Do what works best for you. Include your partner, friends, or anyone who might take care of your baby.

+ Read chapters 11 to 15 for the basics. Read the rest of this chapter about the things you can start getting now.
+ Go to new-parent classes at the hospital or birth center.
+ Watch a video on infant care.
+ Spend time with new moms or dads and their babies.

Breastfeeding your baby

One big decision is about breastfeeding (also called **nursing**). Breastmilk is best for babies. Some families nurse for a few weeks, some nurse for years. Learning about breastfeeding may help you decide if it is right for you.

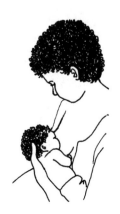

Why is breastfeeding the best choice for many families?

1. Breast milk has everything baby needs in the first six months. As baby gets older, your milk changes, so it's always just right for baby.

Antibodies: Cells made in the body to fight germs. A mom's antibodies get to the baby through breast milk.

2. Only breast milk has antibodies* to protect baby from germs. It can mean baby is less likely to have colds, allergies, ear infections, diarrhea, and other problems.

3. Breastfeeding helps you and your baby feel close. This can be especially helpful when you go back to work. Your baby can drink breast milk by bottle while you're gone. You can still nurse when you and baby are together.

There are lots of great things about breastfeeding. Check out this list of the perks of breastmilk. Mark the ones that help you want to breastfeed.

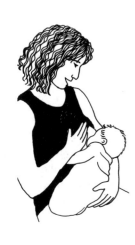

- Breast milk does not cost money.
- It's clean, safe, and ready when you need it. It's the perfect temperature when baby wants to nurse.
- You can feed your baby when they're hungry, almost anywhere you are.
- Breast milk in the first few weeks has extra good stuff in it for baby.
- It has antibodies to help your baby fight germs.
- Even small breasts can make lots of milk.
- Night feedings are often faster and easier when nursing.
- Breastfeeding lets your baby eat just as much as they need. Breastfed babies are less likely to be overweight as they grow up.
- It's something your body likely knows how to do. Even if it takes some time and help, it's an easy way to feed baby for most nursing parents.
- People who breastfeed (or pump their milk) are healthier. Their feelings and their bodies recover from birth faster. Their periods may stay away longer. They're less likely to get cancer, diabetes, and other health problems later in life.

For more on breastfeeding, see chapter 12.

Breastfeeding and working

You can continue to breastfeed after you go back to work. Many nursing parents do this by using a breast pump at work. They take the breast milk home so baby can drink it from a bottle. See chapter 12 for more about pumping milk for your baby.

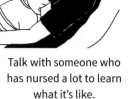

Is nursing right for me?

If you are still not sure you want to breastfeed, take some time. Think about why. Is it something you've heard? Have people tried to talk you out of it? Maybe it's just hard to imagine doing it? Remember, breastfeeding is different for everyone. But it can be hard to try a new thing.

Talk with someone who has nursed a lot to learn what it's like.

Think about all the good things about breastfeeding for both your baby and yourself. Talk to people who have enjoyed breast-feeding. Ask them what helped them get started. Ask how it's been to keep breastfeeding for months or years.

The choice is yours. Only you will know what's right for you and your baby. But, you may not know for sure until you try.

"My best friend told me, 'When I am nursing, I know I'm doing something really special for my baby. Knowing that helps me feel good about myself, even when things are hard."

Feeding your baby formula

Some people can't breastfeed or choose not to. They may have had too much trouble nursing or felt formula was a better fit for them. See chapter 12 to learn more on feeding your baby.

Babies who are not breastfed should always drink formula, NOT plain cow's milk, soy milk, or other kinds of milk. Formula is made to be as much like breast milk as possible. Talk to baby's provider about choosing formula. They can help you know what to look for and what to watch out for. Formula is very expensive. Doctors often have sample cans for you to try. And WIC can help you get formula, too.

Things you and your baby will need

Now's a good time to start thinking about getting clothes, a car seat, and other baby things. It will take time to get all the things your baby needs.

You can get good used clothes and toys from friends, baby gear swaps, and thrift shops. Be careful of secondhand car seats, cribs, and other baby gear. (There is more about secondhand things later in this chapter. Read more about safety in chapter 14.)

Things for baby

☐ **Diapers:** cloth, disposable, or both. Just get one or two packages of newborn diapers, since baby will grow fast. You'll need more of the next size up. Cloth diapers can costs less over time, be gentler on baby's skin, and make less trash. But, they take time to wash. They may be hard to use if you don't have your own washing machine and dryer. Disposables are faster and easier, but cost more and make a lot of trash.

*Onesies: Long shirts that snap at the crotch.

☐ **Warm sleepers with legs, onesies*, socks, a warm hat.** Most babies outgrow the newborn sizes very quickly, unless they're born very small. Get more in sizes 3 to 6 months. A sleep sack can keep baby warm without the risk of blankets in the crib.

*Car seat: A special seat to keep baby safe in motor vehicles. Also called a "car safety seat" or a "child restraint."

☐ **A car seat*** that fits a new baby. Use it on every ride, starting with the trip home from the hospital. This is the law in every state. It's the best thing you can do to protect your baby's life. (More on car seats later in this chapter and in chapter 14.)

☐ **A safe place to sleep,** like a crib or bassinet. It must be sturdy, let baby lie flat, and have a firm mattress that fits snugly. You will want a waterproof pad and a few fitted sheets. (More on safe sleep in chapter 14.)

☐ **Medicine for baby:** Acetaminophen (non-aspirin) baby pain reliever (such as Tylenol) just in case. (DO NOT give ibuprofen to babies less than 6 months old. DO NOT give aspirin to a child of any age.)

☐ **Thermometer:** Get a plain digital thermometer to check for fever. (See chapter 15 for more.)

☐ **First aid kit:** Buy or make a first aid kit with bandages, cleaning wipes, and an ice pack for your home. You can get smaller ones for the car and diaper bag.

Things for you

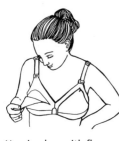

Nursing bra with flaps that open

☐ **Nursing bras:** Start with a stretchy nursing bra or "sleep bra." (These can even help with sore breasts during pregnancy.) After your milk comes in, you might want a more supportive nursing bra. These have cups that open for breastfeeding. Breast pads may help when your breasts leak.

☐ **Breast pump:** If you hope to make milk for baby, it is good to have some kind of breast pump. (It can even help get labor started.) Insurance or WIC may help you get one. See chapter 12 to learn more.

☐ **Bottles and nipples:** If you plan to breastfeed, you may need just a few bottles and nipples for when you pump your breasts. For formula feeding, you will need some newborn formula and at least eight bottles and nipples. Be sure to get some preemie, newborn, or slow-flow nipples.

Other useful things

☐ **A nursing pillow:** a curved pillow that fits around your body on your lap. It helps support baby while nursing.

☐ **A baby tub:** A small plastic bath tub with a sloping back or a foam cushion can help you bathe baby safely.

☐ **A rocking chair:** Rocking in your arms makes many babies feel happy and calm.

☐ **A yoga ball:** Bouncing gently on an exercise ball while you hold her can be very soothing for a new baby. (These are also great in labor!)

☐ **A baby carrier:** Use a cloth baby carrier that holds your baby up high against your chest. It's helpful while doing chores or shopping. It's also great for a fussy baby. Try it on before buying and use it right. (See page 241 for carrier safety.)

☐ **A bouncy seat:** A baby seat that rocks or bounces can calm baby. It is also good to have a safe place to put baby when your arms need a break. Always use the seat harness and keep the seat on the floor. This is not a safe place for baby to sleep for long or be left alone. Many inclined (not flat) baby seats have been recalled.* Always read the instructions and keep baby where you can see them.

$$ Save money: Bed pillows work well for nursing. And a clean sink or a big dishpan makes a good tub while baby is small.

*****Recall:** When it is decided that a product is dangerous and unsafe to keep using. Often happens after babies have died or been hurt while using it. Always check used baby gear for recalls at *cpsc.gov/recalls.*

A one-piece pacifier

☐ **A pacifier:** Sucking can calm a fussy baby. Your breast is best, but a clean finger or baby's own fingers will work, too. Choose a pacifier that is all one piece, with a round nipple. Pacifiers can help keep baby safe while they sleep, but never prop it or force it in. It's important that baby can spit it out if they need to.

☐ **Baby toys:** Rattles, bells, and crinkly things are sounds babies like. Soft, washable toys are good. Toys shouldn't have small parts (like buttons or plastic eyes they could chew off.) If it is small enough to fit in a toilet paper tube, it's a choking hazard for baby. Avoid toys with small batteries, screws, or cords. Remove toys if baby falls asleep.

☐ **Choose colorful things:** Young babies can see bright colors and black and white shapes best.

☐ **Books, handouts, and videos:** Collect information on baby care from your clinic, doctor's office, or bookstore. Look on the internet for more. See chapter 17 for books and websites that are helpful and that you can trust.

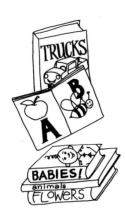

☐ **Picture books:** It's never too early to start reading short picture books to baby. Pick colorful books with words that rhyme.

Choosing the "best" car seat

Riding in a car is one of the most dangerous things we do. A car seat does a very good job of protecting your baby or child in a sudden stop or crash. But make sure you use it right.

There is not one "best" car seat. Try the car seat in your car before you buy it. Make sure it fits and can be tightly installed. If it can't be installed right, take it back. For more about using car seats, see chapter 14.

The best car seat for your new baby:

◆ will fit a small baby by weight and height.

◆ can be used so baby faces the back of the car.

◆ can be buckled tightly in the back seat.

◆ has a harness that's easy to adjust, so you will use it right on every trip.

Kinds of car seats for babies

There are two kinds of car seats you could get for your new baby. Both cover a wide range of weights and ages, so read the labels carefully.

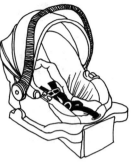

1. **A rear-facing car seat** can only be used rear facing. Most babies will outgrow these (be too tall or too heavy) between 8 and 24 months old. This kind:

   ♦ is easy to carry in and out of the car.

   ♦ often has a base that can stay installed in the car.

   ♦ may be the most useful when baby is small, but he may outgrow it before he is 2 years old. That is when he is old enough to ride forward facing. So you may still have to buy a convertible seat later.

   ♦ may click into a matching stroller.

A rear-facing car seat

2. **A convertible car seat** can be used facing the rear for a baby or toddler. When the child gets too big, the seat can be faced forward. Some convertibles may fit your child all the way until grade school. This kind:

   ♦ Stays secured in the car. You take baby in and out each time you get in and out of the car.

   ♦ Must have a very low shoulder strap setting to fit a new baby well. The more harness settings it has, the longer it will fit your child.

   ♦ Often has higher height and weight limits than a rear-facing only car seat. This means your child can ride rear facing at least two to three years.

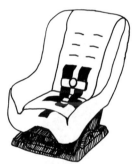

A convertible car seat will give you the best "bang for your buck." It will last the longest.

A more expensive seat is not always safer. All must pass the same tough safety tests. The fit of the car seat in your car and for your baby are most important. There are some great car seats that don't cost a lot and fit new babies well. See chapter 14 for how to find your local car-seat group for help.

If you find it hard to pay for a new car seat, start saving now. Ask your hospital or clinic if they offer low-cost car seats. Find out if your health insurance plan covers car seats. Or, put it on your "wish list" for someone to give as a gift.

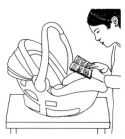

Read the car seat directions to learn how to adjust the harness and install the seat in your car.

Learn how to use the car seat

Get the car seat early. Practice putting a baby doll into the seat. Tighten and loosen the harness. Practice buckling the car seat into your car facing the rear.

Most people don't use their baby's car seats correctly. Mistakes could put your baby in great danger. Follow the car seat and vehicle instructions. Read chapter 14 for details about using a car seat correctly.

Not every car seat fits well in every car. If the one you have does not fit tightly in your car or you have questions, have it checked before the baby comes. Find a trained Child Passenger Safety Technician in your area (see chapter 17).

Choosing secondhand baby gear

Buying all new things for your baby is expensive. Getting some kinds of used baby gear costs less and is good for the Earth. You can find some great deals on baby clothes and toys at yard sales and resale shops. They often look as good as new. You can also find deals on bigger baby gear, but you must make sure it's safe.

Beware: some used things can be dangerous, even if they look safe. Especially things that you put your baby in. Used car seats, cribs, baby carriers, playpens, strollers, and play seats can have serious safety problems. For example, the slats on older cribs were further apart, so babies could get their heads stuck and not be able to breathe.

Problems with used car seats

Try to buy a new car seat, if you can. Old car seats are dangerous. Newer car seats are much safer, even if you don't get a fancy one. See chapter 14 for more about car seats. When looking at a used car seat, find out:

- **Has the car seat been used in a crash?** Most car seat companies say the seats should not be used after any crash, even a small one. It may have hidden damage you can't see. If you don't know its history, don't use it.

- **Does it have its instructions and all its parts?** It's important to follow the instructions because not all car seats work the same way. You can get new instructions or parts from the company (check their website).

- **How old is it?** Check the "expiration" date on the sticker or the back of the car seat. Many companies say not to use car seats more than six years old. A car seat older than 10 years must be thrown away. (Take it apart first, so they can't be found and re-used.)

- **Has the car seat been recalled?** Many recalls are for serious safety hazards. To find out, call the car seat company with the model number and manufacture date or go to _Recalls.gov_. If a used seat doesn't have a sticker with the date and number, there is no way to know it's safe. Don't use it.

Dangers of other used baby gear

Look for the label "JPMA Certified" on any other baby gear you get. Make sure it hasn't been recalled, has all of its parts and instructions, and is in good shape. If you're not sure, don't use it.

Check for baby gear recalls at _cpsc.gov/recalls._

Cribs

Buy a new crib and crib mattress, if you can. There was a big safety update to cribs made after June 2011. If you can't get a new crib, make sure the one you get is safe. Call the company to see if it's been recalled. Make sure the slats (bars) are close enough together that a soda pop can can't go through. It shouldn't have sides that slide down or posts or knobs at the corners.

Playpens or play yards

Don't use a playpen that has been recalled. Make sure the locks on each side work. Get the instructions so you know it's put together right. Playpens with sides that fold down all the way should not be used. (Sides that fold in half and make a "V" are much safer.)

Baby gates

There are gates that bolt into the wall and gates that stay put using pressure. There are gates that open like a door (walk-through) and others that you must step over or take down to get through. Gates for two kinds of openings are:

- **Doorway gates** can be the pressure or bolt kind. Walk-through gates are less likely to cause falls than the kind you step over. If it's a door you go through often, use a walk-through gate.

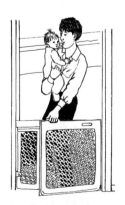

A walk-through gate

- **Stair gates** must be bolted into the wall or railing and must be the walk-through kind. It is too dangerous climb over and risk falling down the stairs.

Look for gates that are smooth on top. Be careful of old folding gates with big diamond-shaped holes. They can strangle a baby.

For product safety and recall resources, see chapter 17.

Tips for partners

- Learn about birth. Go to birth classes together.
- If you don't think you want to be the birth partner, be honest.
- Learn about baby care.
- Take parental leave if you can. It will help you bond with baby. Talk with your boss.
- Do what you can to support your partner's desire to breastfeed as long as they want to.
- Help choose a car seat. Learn how to install it in the back seat. Go to a car seat check to make sure you've got it right.
- Help get baby's gear ready. Put together the crib. Learn how to use your baby carrier.

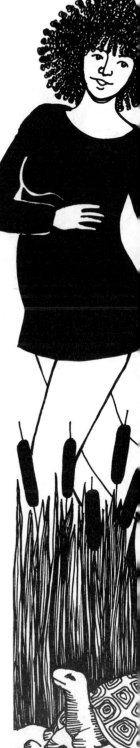

Your First Trimester

The nine months of pregnancy are divided into "trimesters." In this book, each trimester has its own chapter. It starts with how your baby and body are changing. Then it covers other important things to know or think about at that time. At the end, you can fill-in notes from your checkup. It's also a good place to write down questions you want to ask.

Trimesters, months, and weeks

Many people think about the months of pregnancy. However, your provider may talk about it in weeks. This is because your unborn baby grows so much during each week. There will be about 40 weeks from the start of your last period until your baby's birth.

This is how the weeks and months are divided up:

1st trimester = weeks 1 through 13

2nd trimester = weeks 14 through 27

3rd trimester = weeks 28 through 40

You will feel different in each trimester. At first, you may be uncomfortable as your body gets used to being pregnant. In the second trimester, you will probably feel more comfortable. Pregnancy may seem easier.

In the third trimester, you may have more aches and pains. As your uterus gets really big, it pushes against other organs. Your hips and pelvis get ready for birth. You may wish that baby would come soon. However, the longer baby stays inside, the better.

How your body changes as your baby grows

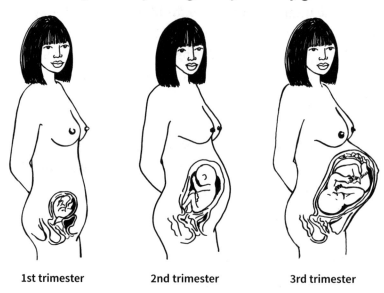

1st trimester　　　　　2nd trimester　　　　　3rd trimester

Main things to keep in mind

You've learned so much about caring for your body and your baby. Look back on chapters 2 through 6 as much as you like. The biggest things to remember are:

- Go to all of your prenatal visits.
- Learn about pregnancy, birth, postpartum, and baby care from people, books, and websites you trust.

♦ Talk to your partner or your loved ones about how you're feeling. If you feel depressed, tell someone.

♦ Call your doctor, midwife, or nurse if you ever feel that something is wrong in your body.

At prenatal visits, your provider will look at how baby is growing. He'll also check your health. These visits are the best time for you to ask questions. They also help the provider get to know you. You should also get to meet the other doctors or midwives who may care for you when your provider is out.

Your regular checkups will include:

♦ weight.

♦ temperature.

♦ blood pressure.

♦ lungs.

♦ breasts.

♦ uterus size.

♦ baby's heartbeat (starting in the fourth month).

As your pregnancy goes along, your provider will use ultrasound to look at the baby's growth, the placenta, and the uterus. Usually, you and your partner will be able to see the ultrasound screen. You may be able to get a printed picture of the baby. If you want to know if your baby is a boy or girl, he will use ultrasound to find out. If you don't want to know, be sure to tell them before ultrasounds.

Your provider will check your blood type. They will also test your blood and urine for any problems, such as anemia, diabetes, and infections. If a test is positive, they will run more tests. If there is a problem, they will talk with you about how to take care of it. Remember, you can always ask questions.

Weeks 1 through 13

The first few months of pregnancy are very different for everyone. Some people don't tell others they're pregnant yet. Some don't look or feel pregnant yet. Others feel it at the very beginning and tell people right away. No matter how you feel in these first months, there are amazing things going on inside of you.

Your baby in your body

Look at the picture below. Your unborn baby lives in your **uterus**. They are curled up in the **amniotic sac** (bag of waters) filled with **amniotic fluid (water).**

Baby's **umbilical cord** is attached to the placenta. The **placenta** is attached to the inside of your uterus. The blood in the placenta and cord carries food and oxygen from you to your baby. It can also carry things that could harm your baby, like alcohol or nicotine. The placenta takes waste away from your baby's blood.

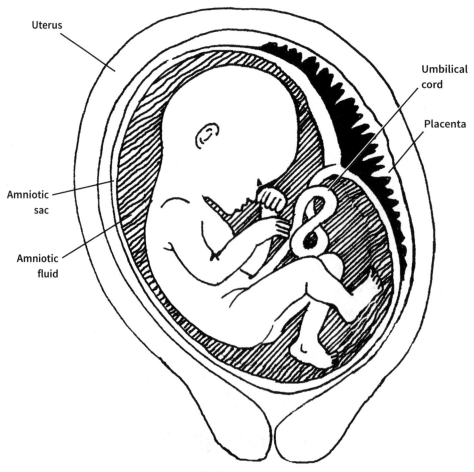

Your baby's home in your uterus

How your baby is growing

In the first month, the fertilized egg looks kind of like a raspberry. Its cells will turn into your baby and the placenta.

Weeks 5 through 8

In the second month, your baby starts taking shape. The placenta gives baby food, oxygen, and hormones. They will grow to be about 1/2-inch long (half the size of a quarter!).

By the end of week 8:

- baby has the cells that will form her skin, nervous system, bones, muscles, heart, and other organs.
- their neural tube is longer and closes (this is the start of their brain and spinal cord)
- their head has the start of eyes, ears, nose, mouth, and nostrils.
- they have small paddles that will turn into arms, legs, and tiny webbed fingers and toes.

Weeks 9 through 13

Baby changes quickly in this last month. They will grow to be 2–3 inches long and weigh about 1/2 an ounce. By the end of week 13, baby's:

- bones are longer and stronger.
- fingernails are growing.
- skin is thin and see-through.
- genitals start to form.
- kidneys start making urine (pee).
- eyelids form but are closed.

How your body is changing

Weeks 1 through 8

- About two weeks after your period starts, your egg and the sperm come together through sex or fertility help. This is conception, the start of your baby.

- You will have no period about two weeks after conception. The fertilized egg attaches to the wall of your uterus.
- You may start feeling sick to your stomach (nauseous) and tired.
- Your breasts may start to feel full and may get sore. Your nipples may start to get darker.
- Your skin may feel dry or have more pimples than usual.
- You may get a dark line down the center of your belly.

Weeks 9 through 13

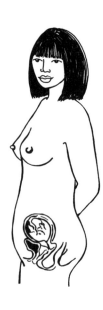

- You may be starting to gain weight. By the end of this month, you probably will have gained 2 to 5 pounds (1 to 2.25 kg). You may need some bigger clothes soon.
- Your breasts may feel very heavy. This is normal. You may need bigger bras that fit well.
- By the end of this month, you may be able to feel your growing uterus. Push gently on your belly, just above your pubic hair. Your uterus will feel firm and round, like an orange.
- You may get constipated more often than before. Eat plenty of fiber, especially fruit, whole grains, and bran. Drink a lot of water, too. Ask your provider before taking any medicine for constipation.

Taking care of yourself

Start taking care of yourself right away! Some of your baby's most important growth happens in these first months. Follow the healthy habits in chapters 2 and 3.

How much weight should I gain?

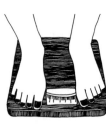

It's important to eat enough during pregnancy. But, you shouldn't eat twice as much as before you got pregnant. Most people need to eat only a little more than normal while pregnant. Be sure to eat healthy foods and take prenatal vitamins. You and your baby need the best nutrition possible. See chapter 4 for more about healthy foods.

Healthy weight gain is different for everyone

How much to gain depends on your weight and health before you got pregnant. Talk with your doctor or midwife about what's healthy for you. Gaining too much or too little weight is not healthy. It can cause serious problems for both you and baby.

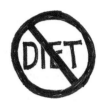

A note on eating disorders

If you have had problems with healthy eating, tell your provider. Eating disorders can be very hard while pregnant. The fear of getting bigger and the stress of knowing your baby needs you to eat is a lot to cope with.

If you have fears about food or weight gain, your provider can help. They may talk with a dietitian (healthy-eating specialist) to help make a food plan that is good for you and baby.

A note for teens

If you're a teenager, remember that your own body is still growing, too. It's very important to eat enough for you and the baby. Eat well and skip the junk food. Your provider can help you figure out what's right for you.

Stay healthy

+ Go to your prenatal visits. Learn about pregnancy.
+ Eat the healthy foods that you and your baby need. Take your prenatal vitamins every day.
+ Get plenty of rest. Take time to sit down, take deep breaths, and relax.
+ Get some exercise every day. Walk instead of driving when you can. Take the stairs instead of the elevator at work. Park far from the door when you go shopping.
+ Drink lots of water. Skip the sodas and energy drinks. Slices of fruit or cucumber mixed with sparkling water makes a yummy drink.
+ Floss and brush your teeth and gums. Go to the dentist and get any problems treated. Tell them you are pregnant.

Warning Signs – Emergency

Learn these warning signs of health problems during pregnancy. Call your health care provider if you think you might have any of them.

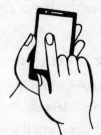

- ◆ Bleeding from your vagina
- ◆ Sudden swelling of your face, hands, feet
- ◆ Dizziness
- ◆ Trouble seeing
- ◆ Bad headaches
- ◆ Pain or cramping in your belly
- ◆ Pain while urinating (peeing)
- ◆ Thoughts of harming yourself or the baby

Stay safe

- ◆ Don't use tobacco, alcohol, or drugs. Stay away from places where others are smoking or using. Ask people not to smoke in your car or home.
- ◆ Wear your seat belt on every car ride.
- ◆ Protect yourself from STDs if you or your partner have sex with other people.
- ◆ Ask your provider or a pharmacist before taking any medicines. Tell them you are pregnant.

Why am I so tired?

In the first few months, you may feel very tired. Growing a baby is hard work for your body! Eating well, exercising, and getting more sleep will give you more energy. Take naps and go to bed a bit earlier than normal. If you want to rest, learn to say "no" to friends who want to go out. Your energy will come back in the next trimester.

What can I do if my stomach is upset?

In the first two or three months, you may feel like throwing up often. You may even vomit daily. This is called **morning sickness** but it can happen at any time of day. It usually stops after the first trimester. Here are some things that may help:

- Eat small meals every two or three hours. Don't wait until you feel really hungry. Bring snacks with you when you go out. Eat a small snack before going to bed.

- Keep some plain crackers next to your bed. Eat a few crackers before getting up in the morning or when you start to feel sick.

- Sip a little fizzy water or ginger ale.

- Eat only the food that you feel hungry for. Don't worry right now if it's not the most nutritious. Eat what you can keep down. You can eat healthy foods when you feel better.

- Stop eating foods that make you feel sick, especially greasy or spicy foods.

- After you vomit, wait a few hours before eating. Then start with water or weak tea with a little sugar. This gives your body back the liquid it has lost.

- Vitamin pills could upset your stomach if you haven't been eating. Try taking them with food. Or try to take them before you go to bed, so you can sleep through any burps.

"Adding a piece of fresh ginger to my water really calmed my tummy."

After you vomit, rinse your mouth with baking soda mixed with water. Then spit it out. This keeps the acid in vomit from hurting your teeth.

Sometimes the smells or sounds around you make you feel sick. Stress, anger, and worry can also make it worse. Talk to your partner, friends, and family. Tell them how you're feeling and how they can help you. They may not know that their perfume, smelly food, or loud music is making you sick.

If you're vomiting every day, call your provider. Also call if you get dizzy or pass out. They can try to help and make sure your body has enough fluids.

Why do my moods change so much?

In the first few months, your moods are will likely to go up and down like a roller coaster. This is very normal. It is from hormones changing in early pregnancy. Your moods should calm down after month three.

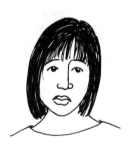

You may have fears or worries about birth or your baby's health. This is normal, too. Sharing your thoughts can help. Learning more may make you less afraid.

- *I'm worried that my baby won't be normal.* Most babies are born healthy. You will have tests during pregnancy to find some of the rare problems a baby might have. Ask your provider about these tests. Meanwhile, do what you can to have a healthy baby.

- *I'm scared of what labor will be like.* A childbirth class will help you know what to expect. You'll also learn ways to cope with pain. You can also read and watch videos about birth. (See chapter 10 and use resources in chapter 17.)

- *What if I'm not a good parent?* It's normal to worry that you might not be the best parent. Remember that everyone has to learn how to be a good parent. You can practice by helping to care for a friend's baby. Talk to other parents about what it's been like for them.

Things to do to help yourself feel better

- Cook a healthy and delicious meal that you love.

- Take a walk every day. Going with a friend can be more fun than going alone. It also gives you time to visit.

- Try learning something new, like how to crochet. You could make a hat for your baby.

- Do something nice for someone, like babysitting for a friend or visiting an elderly neighbor.

- Have a fun night out with your friends. See a feel-good movie or play a game that makes you laugh.

- Ask your partner to rub your neck or feet.

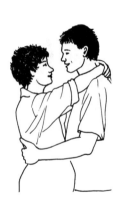

Talking about feelings can help

If you are feeling blue, tell someone who cares about you! This might be your partner, your mom, sister, or friend. Choose people who will really listen and don't try to tell you what to do. Just talking can help you feel a lot better.

Who would you talk to if you were upset?

1. _____

2. _____

3. _____

How do you feel now?

_____

_____

_____

_____

What worries do you have?

_____

_____

_____

_____

What makes you feel happy now?

_____

_____

_____

_____

If it gets to be too much

For many pregnant people these strong emotions and worries can lead to depression* and anxiety** during pregnancy and after. If you or a family member has had mental health problems, you are at higher risk while pregnant. It can affect your health and your baby's, but you don't have to suffer.

*Depression: A mood illness (disorder) that causes sadness or loss of interest.

Go to page 278 to learn about mood disorders and how to tell if that's what's going on for you. If you're not sure, go to page 291 to figure out what kind of help you need right now. Chapter 17 has lists of programs that can offer support by phone, text, and online. You don't have to do this alone.

**Anxiety (ang-zy-e-tee): A mood disorder that causes strong worry, fear, or panic.

If you need help right now, call or text 9-8-8

Facts about partner abuse

For some people, home isn't a safe place. Partners may hit, beat, control, or yell at them. Even if they only shout or call names, it can hurt. This abuse often starts or gets worse during pregnancy.

Domestic violence is a crime. It also is a serious health problem that hurts mom, baby, and other kids in the home.

If this is happening to you, you may feel ashamed. But you're not to blame. The person who hurts you is the one who is wrong.

If you're being abused, you don't need to take it!

There is help for you

- Call the free national hotline (below). It can give you information and local contacts for shelters, counseling, and legal help.
- Tell a trusted friend, doctor or nurse, clergy member, or counselor.
- Learn about safe places to go if you need to leave your home. There are shelters that can hide you and give you protection.

If you think a friend is being abused

Do you know someone who fears their partner? People often hide signs of abuse. A few signs to look for are:

- Bruises or other injuries they blame on "accidents"
- Staying home alone most of the time
- Increased alcohol or drug use

Share the free hotline number shown to the right. Encourage your friend to get help. It can be very hard for someone to take steps to protect themselves on their own.

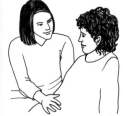

National Domestic Violence Hotline, 800-799-7233

Common worries

Could I be having twins or multiples?*

Twins are not very likely. More than two are very rare. If your mom is a fraternal twin (not identical), you are more likely to have twins. Identical twins happen only by chance.

Tests can be done to check the number of embryos early in pregnancy. Usually they can be seen in ultrasounds.

If you are having twins or more, there are some extra risks. Your provider will talk with you about the special care you may need. With good care and healthy habits, you are very likely to have healthy babies.

Things that may happen with twins or multiples. You may:

* gain more weight than with a single baby.
* need more rest (lying on your left side is best).
* have more checkups later in pregnancy.
* go into preterm labor (see chapter 8).
* need a c-section.

*Multiples: Two or more babies.

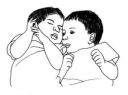

Twins love to be close to each other, like they were in the womb.

Could I lose my baby? – Miscarriage

When a pregnancy ends on its own before the 20th week, it is called a miscarriage. People may not talk about it, but miscarriage is very common. Most are caused by things you had no control over. Many losses happen due to problems with the cells as they try to form a baby. They are not caused by things you do in your daily life, like feeling stressed, getting exercise, or having sex.

Warning signs of miscarriage

Know how to reach your doctor, midwife, or nurse at all hours. Call if any of these things happen:

* Bleeding from your vagina
* Painful cramps in your belly or back
* A jelly-like blob coming from your vagina. (If this happens, save it in a plastic bag for them to see.)

Some health problems, germs, and infections make miscarriage more likely. So can some drugs, alcohol, and some chemicals. Severe injury or abuse can also put baby at risk. Go back to chapters 3 and 4 to learn more about risks. Talk to your provider about ways to help keep you and your baby healthy and safe.

How do I know if I'm having a miscarriage?

If it happens in the first month, it may just seem like a heavy period that came late. You may not even have known you were pregnant. If it happens later, you will have more bleeding and cramps. You may have red tissue blobs (blood clots) come out of your vagina. They may be small or as big as a lemon. If you are more than two months along, you may see the forming baby in one of these clots.

What do I do if I think I'm losing the baby?

Many miscarriages. Be sure to tell your provider if you have had more than one miscarriage. This can help them know how to best help you have a healthy pregnancy.

Call your provider right away. Tell them what's happening and why you're worried. If you are still in the early weeks, they might tell you to wait and see. If you are more than a month along, they may want you to come in. They may offer medicine to help things pass more quickly. The more weeks along you are, they may offer a procedure that uses gentle suction to get all of the tissue out. Miscarriages can be dangerous if not treated. Your provider can help you choose what is best for you.

After a miscarriage

Call the All-Options Talkline for support during or after pregnancy loss at (1-888-493-0092).

Once your body has been taken care of after a miscarriage, you may be left with some very hard feelings. You may be very sad for weeks or even months. You may feel guilty that you feel relieved that you're not pregnant. You may feel like you did something wrong. All of these feelings are normal, but they are also very hard. It can help to talk to someone who knows what you're going through. Tell your provider how you feel. Ask them what you should know about getting pregnant again. Or, ask about birth control to prevent it until you're ready. Take care of yourself as you heal.

Prenatal testing

There are a lot of tests done early in pregnancy. These tests help your provider take good care of you. They also help you plan for any special care your baby may need later.

Routine (common) tests

Blood draw	A needle is used to take some of your blood, commonly from your arm. This blood is used to look for signs of illness or health problems. It is also used to check your blood type and *Rh factor**.
Urinalysis (urine sample)	A sample of your urine is tested for signs of problems or infection. Your provider will give you simple instructions with a clean sample cup for you to use in the restroom.

Rh: A protein in blood. Rh+ (Rh positive) blood has this protein. Rh– (Rh negative) blood does not. If your blood is Rh–, it can make antibodies that will severely harm your baby. To prevent this, you will need a medicine called Rh immunoglobulin (RhIg). You may need it again after birth.

Your provider will ask what vaccines you have had. They'll also ask if you have ever had the measles or chickenpox. If you haven't done it already, they will want to test for hepatitis, HIV, and other STIs. If any tests come back positive, your provider will help you decide how to treat them and how to protect baby.

Genetic tests

Some babies are born with a health condition that started while their cells were still forming. This is called a **birth defect**. Some birth defects are serious, but some are not. Some can be found before birth, but some cannot.

How can I find out if my baby will have a birth defect?

The first step is to tell your provider about any birth defects or genetic diseases that you know of in your or your partner's family. They may help you find a genetic counselor to figure out baby's risk.

If someone in your or your partner's family had a birth defect, tell your provider. They can help you find a genetic counselor to talk with about your baby's risk.

Screens vs. diagnostic tests

Screening tests tell you how likely it is that your baby is at risk for the most common birth defects. Screens are done on one or both parents, by blood test or cheek swab. There is no risk to you or baby.

Diagnostic tests tell you if your baby has one of the more common genetic birth defects. These tests are done using cells from placenta tissue or amniotic fluid, which both have some of baby's cells in them.

First trimester screening	A blood test ("maternal screen") and ultrasound to check for risk of things like Down syndrome or heart defects. Done during weeks 10 to 13.
Carrier screening	A blood test or mouth swab to see if either parent carries the genes for certain genetic diseases, such as cystic fibrosis or sickle cell disease. Done anytime.
Cell-free DNA testing—also called NIPT (screening)	A test using your blood to check baby's DNA for genetic defects. Done during week 10 or later.
Chorionic villus sampling (diagnostic)	A tiny bit of tissue is taken from the placenta. These cells are tested for genetic defects. Cramping is common, small risk of bleeding or infection. Very small risk of miscarriage. Done during weeks 10 to 13.

Should I have these tests? Or wait?

This is your choice. Talk to your provider about what feels right to you. Some questions you might ask are:

+ *What will it tell us?*
+ *Is it painful or risky?*
+ *What if the test is positive?*
+ *What if I don't do it?*
+ *Is it covered by insurance?*

"I did it so I could have time to learn about my baby's needs. I wanted time to prepare myself."

Many people choose to have these tests done early while they can still choose whether or not to stay pregnant.

Others choose to wait and do a combined screening and/or diagnostic test in the second trimester. Those tests tell you more and have a little less risk, but they are done later. See chapter 8 to learn more.

After birth, all babies born in the US are also screened for genetic problems. These are rare but serious, so early screening is important so baby can get the best care right away. See chapter 11 for more on newborn screenings.

Keeping up your healthy habits

How are you doing? You probably have been making some big changes in your life and activities. Many people must work hard to change how they eat, sleep, or exercise while pregnant.

An exercise to do now: The bridge

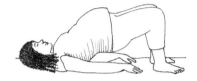

It's never too soon to start making your tummy muscles and back stronger. Look back at chapter 3 to review the exercises there.

Bridge can make your tummy, back, and shoulders feel really good. Lie on your back with your knees bent. Breathe out and push with your legs to raise your bottom and back off the floor slowly. Breathe in. Then breathe out and tighten your tummy while you roll your back and bottom back to the floor slowly. Breathe in while you lie flat. Then do it again five or ten times.

It's hard to change habits

You know that smoking, drinking alcohol, or taking drugs can harm your baby. Quitting is not always easy. If you need help breaking bad habits, ask for it. Talk with your provider about getting help. There are programs to help people quit smoking, drinking, or using.

Starting new healthy habits isn't easy either. Your partner, friends, and family will want to help. But, you may have to tell them what you need.

What's been the hardest to change?

_____

_____

_____

What's been the easiest to change?

_____

_____

_____

Who's helping you make changes?

_____

_____

_____

_____

What healthy habits are you still working on?

_____

_____

_____

_____

Tips for partners

- Be ready for your partner to be more emotional than usual. Try to go with the ups and downs.

- Your partner may feel much more tired than usual. Their body is working hard—be patient and kind.

- Help out where you can. Take on some of their chores or ask how you can help.

- Offer to go along for checkups or tests. Make sure both you and your partner's questions are answered.

- If a miscarriage happens, you may both feel the loss. Talk to your partner, even when it's hard. Listen to their feelings, even if they don't make sense to you.

   Saying you're sorry is often better than saying they can have more babies.

   Remember, most miscarriages do not happen because of something either parent did wrong.

Monthly checkups

All about me (things to tell your provider)

I am _____ years old. My birthday is _____.
(month, day, year)

I am _____ inches tall and weighed _____ pounds/kg before I got pregnant.

My last period started on _____.
(date)

- Health problems I have (illnesses, surgeries, etc.):

  _____

  _____

  _____

- Health problems in my family, my partner, my other children, my parents, brothers, sisters:

  _____

  _____

  _____

- Medicines, herbs, and supplements I use:

  _____

  _____

  _____

- Questions I have about being pregnant:

  _____

  _____

  _____

First prenatal checkup notes

(Write down what happens at each checkup to help you remember.)

Date _____ (usually 4 to 8 weeks after your last period)

I am about _____ weeks pregnant today.

I weigh _____ pounds/kg.

My blood pressure is _____/_____.

Tests I had today:

_____

_____

_____

My provider's name is

_____

Phone number:_____

Emergency phone number:_____

Email address: _____

Things I learned today:

1. My baby's "due date": _____

_____

2. _____

_____

_____

3. _____

_____

_____

My next checkup will be on

The _____ of _____, at _____:_____.
    (date)   **(month)**   **(time)**

Your first visit is often longer than the rest. In shorter visits, it is easy to forget what you wanted to talk about. Write down your worries or questions to bring with you at each checkup. Make notes about what your provider says.

If you **do not want to know the sex of the baby**, ask your provider to write that in your chart. Remind them at the start of each checkup and each ultrasound.

Questions you may want to ask at your next checkup

- ◆ *What can I do if I am constipated?*
- ◆ *Why do I feel so happy one day and so sad the next?*
- ◆ *Am I gaining enough weight?*

Questions I have:

1._____

2._____

3._____

Prenatal checkup notes

On this date, _____, I had my second visit.

I am _____ weeks pregnant.

I weigh _____ pounds/kg now.

I have gained _____ pounds/kg since my last checkup.

My blood pressure is _____/_____.

Things I learned today:

1. _____

_____

2. _____

_____

3. _____

_____

My next checkup will be on

The _____ of _____, at _____:_____.

(date)   (month)   (time)

Questions for next time:

1._____

2._____

3._____

4._____

Prenatal checkup notes

On this date, _____, I had my second visit.

I am _____ weeks pregnant.

I weigh _____ pounds/kg now.

I have gained _____ pounds/kg since my last checkup.

My blood pressure is _____/_____.

Things I learned today:

1. _____

_____

2. _____

_____

3. _____

_____

My next checkup will be on

The _____ of _____, at _____:_____.
     (date)   (month)   (time)

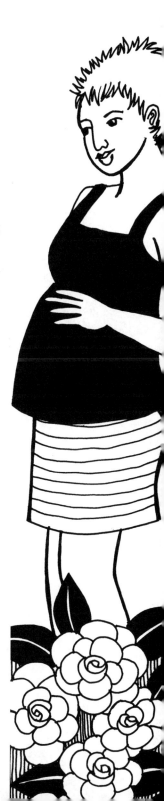

Chapter 8

Your Second Trimester

Weeks 14 through 27

Your body is getting used to having a baby growing inside. You probably will feel better in this trimester than before. You may have more energy and less morning sickness.

Your body will really change shape now. Exercise becomes more and more important. Strengthen your back and belly to hold your growing baby.

It can be very exciting to feel the baby move. At 20 weeks, you are half-way through your pregnancy. Now is the time to sign up for a childbirth class. Take one that will end before your ninth month starts.

Look in this chapter for:

How your baby is growing

Weeks 14 through 17

In the fourth month, baby starts to look much more like a baby! They may be close to five inches long and weigh over four ounces. By the end of week 17, baby's:

- genitals will be formed enough to see.
- neck can hold hold up their head and their eyes can slowly move.
- fingers and toes are well formed. Even the toenails!
- fine hair is starting to grow.
- arms and legs can move enough to see on ultrasound, but not to feel just yet.
- organs are working hard to make and pump lots of blood.

Weeks 18 through 21

This month means you are halfway through your pregnancy! You will start to feel your baby moving very soon. They will grow to be over 6 inches long and weight more than 11 ounces. By the end of week 21, baby's:

- ears start sticking out and they can hear sounds.
- organs are working well and their first poop starts forming.
- skin is covered with a thick cream called *vernix* to keep it healthy.
- skin has tiny hairs called *lanugo* to help hold the vernix on.
- (in females) uterus, vagina, and ovaries (with eggs!) grow.
- able to suck their thumb.

Weeks 22 through 27

Your baby is growing details for the rest of this trimester. They may be more than nine inches long and weigh around two pounds. By the end of week 27, baby's:

- hair and eyebrows can be seen.
- skin is pink and wrinkly.

- moving when they hear your voice or a loud noise. Baby has asleep and awake times that you can feel.
- kicks and flips are strong. You may even feel his hiccups!
- lungs are making a slimy coating inside to help them work.

How your body is changing

Weeks 14 through 17

- You are starting to gain weight more quickly. Ask your provider how much is healthy for you to gain each week.
- Morning sickness will likely end. You will start to feel hungry more often.
- Your breasts may be less sore than before.
- You may not need to go to the bathroom as often.
- You might feel your baby move, like a little flutter or a gas bubble. If not, don't worry. It's still early.
- Your belly starts to show and you may need to wear bigger clothes and bras.
- You may feel dizzy if you move quickly. Be sure to drink lots of water. Sit up for a moment before standing to make sure you feel steady.

Weeks 18 through 21

- By week 20 you should feel your baby move often. If not, tell your provider.
- The top of your uterus may be up to your belly button.
- Your face may get light or dark patches. A dark line may run down the middle of your belly. These changes should go away after your baby is born.
- You may have pains in your sides, hips, and thighs from your growing belly.
- You may have some swelling and tingling in your hands and feet.

Weeks 22 through 27

- The top of your uterus is now above your belly button.
- The skin on your belly, breasts, hands, and feet may itch.
- You may start to feel your uterus contracting and relaxing.
- You may get stretch marks on your belly and breasts.
- Your belly button may pop out.
- Your legs may get cramps and your ankles may swell.
- The areolas around your nipples may look bigger and darker.

Tuning up your body for life

Our bodies are made for moving, not sitting still. When you are active, you help your muscles. Remember this when you are reaching up to a high shelf or sweeping the floor.

If you have to sit most of the day at work, get up every hour for just a few minutes. Move around, even if you stay at your desk. Walk while you talk on the phone. If you are watching TV, get up during commercials. Moving around is one of the best healthy habits to do throughout your life.

Walking for health

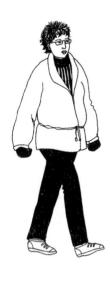

- Take a half-hour walk every day. You don't have to do it all at once. Wear comfortable sport shoes. For the best workout, go fast, but not so fast that you can't talk. Swing your arms to exercise your upper body.
- Take walks in different places so you don't get bored. Invite a friend to the mall or a park. When you walk alone, listen to music or a book.
- Walk tall. Hold your belly in and your shoulders back.

Exercises to help you get ready for birth

Birth will be easier if you are in good shape. Remember the exercises in chapter 3. They will help your core to be strong for birth. Here are some more to do every day.

Kegel squeeze helps hold up your uterus

This exercise strengthens the muscles around your vagina. These muscles help hold up the weight of your baby and uterus. They also help you control your urine (pee). After birth, the Kegel squeeze helps keep your vagina and bladder strong. This exercise will help you even as you get older.

An easy way to learn to do the Kegel squeeze is while you are peeing on the toilet. Here's how:

1. Squeeze the muscles you use to stop your pee. These are muscles around your vagina and perineum*. This is called the Kegel squeeze. Try **not** to use your stomach muscles or buttocks.

   *Perineum: The skin and tissue between the vagina and anus.

2. Hold tight while you count 1–2–3–4–5.

3. Relax, and then squeeze again. (Once you know how this exercise feels, don't do it on the toilet.)

You can do Kegels anywhere. Try it standing at the kitchen sink or waiting for the bus. Practice until you can do it 25 times, three or four times a day.

Squats help strengthen your core

Squatting strengthens your tummy, legs, and back. It also stretches your hips and the joints of your pelvis. Being able to squat helps a lot when you carry the extra weight of your baby inside. The stretching will help baby come through the birth canal.

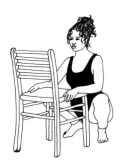

Squat holding onto a chair for balance.

Here's how to practice squatting:

1. Stand facing a chair with feet apart.

2. Pull your tummy in and keep your back as straight as possible.

3. Bend your knees and squat down slowly, holding onto the chair. (Don't do this if your knees hurt.)

4. Rise up slowly, keeping your shoulders back.

5. Do this slowly 5 or 10 times.

Learning to lift safely

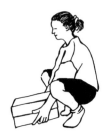

Lifting safely by squatting with back straight.

Learning to squat will protect your back later. It is the safest way to lift heavy things. You will be doing a lot of lifting as your baby grows.

Sitting with knees spread

Stretching helps you spread your hips and knees wide apart during birth. Here's an easy way to stretch while you are relaxing:

1. Sit on the floor with your back straight.

2. Put the soles of your feet together.

3. Spread your knees wide apart and keep them there for a minute or two.

4. Pull your knees together, then spread them wide again.

Healthy snacks to remember

- **Fresh fruits**—orange, apple, peach, or papaya with non-fat, non-sweetened yogurt on top. Add chopped walnuts for crunch.

- **Trail mix**—raisins, apricots, or prunes mixed with pumpkin seeds, peanuts, or almonds.

- **Raw vegetables**—carrots, tomatoes, or broccoli to dip in hummus or yogurt.

- **Whole grains**—bread or crackers with peanut butter.

- **Water**—instead of sodas or too much coffee.

Keeping that loving feeling

Having sex is safe and healthy in a normal pregnancy. Your provider will tell you not to have sex if there is reason to worry.

The changes happening to you can mean sex and intimacy feel different. Some people feel very sexy while pregnant. Others don't want to have sex at all.

Tell your partner how you're feeling. Ask what he or she is feeling, too. There are many ways to enjoy sex. Talk about what you think might feel good. Try different positions, like you being on top or lying on your side with your partner behind you. Or, using hands or mouths might be more comfortable. Try other ways of being close, like cuddling or massaging each other.

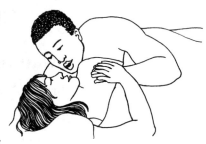

If you don't want to have sex, or it doesn't feel good, say so. If it is hard for you or your partner to not have sex, try to remind each other that it won't last forever.

When you do have sex, it is safest for you and baby if you only have sex with someone who is only having sex with you. Be sure to use a condom if either of you has had sex with someone else. That will help prevent you from getting an infection that could hurt your baby. If any fluid or blood comes from your vagina, stop having sex and call your provider right away.

Spending time with older children

If you have other kids, make sure you spend time with them. Talk about the baby who is coming. Read some books together about new babies. Give both boys and girls a doll so they will have their own baby. All these things will help make this big change seem more real. Let them know that you will still love them after the baby is born. Some practical tips:

- ◆ If you plan to move a child's bed into a different room, do it a few months before the baby is born.

- ◆ Get a few new clothes, books, and toys for them. That way, they can have some special things just for them after baby comes.

Help for common problems

How to cool heartburn

*Heartburn:
Sharp or burning
chest pains from acid
backing up into the
tube that goes from
your mouth to your
stomach.

Heartburn* after eating is common in pregnancy. These tips
might help you feel better:

- Eat smaller meals, more often.

- Chew your food well.

- Stop eating foods that make it worse. Spicy or greasy foods
  are common causes.

- Wait one to three hours after eating to go to bed.

- Lie down with your head and back propped up a bit.

- Wear clothes that are loose around your waist.

If these things don't work, ask your provider what medicines
you can take safely to help you feel better.

How to avoid swollen feet and ankles

Are your ankles and feet swollen? Some swelling is normal in
pregnancy. You should keep drinking plenty of water. Here are
some other ways to help:

- Wear support hose and shoes with low heels.

- Lie on the bed with your legs higher that your head. Put
  your feet up against the wall or up on pillows.

- Move your legs often, pointing your toes, and making
  circles with your feet.

- Put one foot up on a low stool or box when you have to
  stand.

- Sleep on your left side.

- Stay away from salty foods, caffeine, and diet sodas.

- Swim or do exercises in a swimming pool.

Sudden swelling is a warning sign. Call your provider right away.

How to deal with varicose veins

Many people get swollen blue (varicose) veins during pregnancy. These veins are most common in your legs, but can also happen around your vagina. Varicose veins are often painless, but can get quite sore. Here are ways to prevent them or keep them from getting worse. They usually go away a little while after baby is born.

- ◆ Walk every day. Exercising your leg muscles helps keep the blood flowing well in your veins.
- ◆ Put your feet up when you sit down.
- ◆ Take breaks and change position often when you sit or stand for a long time.
- ◆ Wear support hose and comfortable shoes.

If you have varicose veins around your vagina, ask your provider about getting a special sling (support garment).

How to deal with hemorrhoids

Hemorroids are swollen veins in your anus and rectum that can itch, hurt, or bleed. They often can get worse if you often have to strain (push hard) to have bowel movements.

To feel better, wipe the area with witch hazel* pads. Soaking in a warm bath can also feel good. Talk to your provider if you think you have hemorrhoids.

The best way to keep from having hemorrhoids is to keep your stools (poop) soft. (See below for tips on preventing constipation.)

*Witch hazel:
A soothing, safe natural remedy available at drug stores. It comes in a bottle or on pads.

Are your nipples shaped right for breastfeeding?

If your nipples don't stick out, you don't need to worry. You can still breastfeed.

Some nipples are flat. Try squeezing them around the edge of the areola (dark area). If they do not stick out more when you squeeze, they are inverted.

Some nipples stick out more as pregnancy goes on. If they do not, there are simple things to do when you start breastfeeding. You

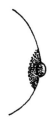

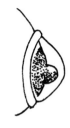

Nipple shell

can use a device to pull out the nipple. Your nurse or breastfeeding consultant can help you get started.

How can you relieve breast pain?

As your breasts get bigger and heavier, they may hurt. A bra that fits well will keep them as comfortable as possible. You may want a stronger bra for during the day and a stretchy bra to wear at home or at night.

How can you cope with constipation*?

*Constipation: Bowel movements that don't come at least every two or three days. They are very dry and hard.

Constipation is very uncomfortable during pregnancy. Here are some tips to keep stools soft:

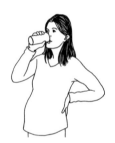

- ◆ Exercise every day.
- ◆ Drink eight to twelve tall glasses of liquids every day; at least half should be water.
- ◆ Eat foods with lots of fiber, such as fresh fruits and vegetables, whole grain cereal and bread, and beans.
- ◆ Snack on dried prunes or apricots each day.
- ◆ Get plenty of rest and time with loved ones. Stress and worry can make constipation worse.

If you get constipated often, try drinking warm prune juice. Ask your provider if you should take extra fiber or a stool softener.

Prenatal testing

Your baby's body has grown so much! Their brain, nervous system, and organs are mostly working. This means that testing done now can tell you a lot more than early on.

Routine tests

An **ultrasound** is often done in the second trimester to see how baby is growing. They will look at and measure baby's body parts and organs. They will also check the position of the placenta and the uterus. This information can tell your provider if there is a risk of problems in labor. It can often also tell you the sex of the baby, if you want to know. (If you don't want to know, be sure to tell them before the ultrasound!)

Ultrasound (sonogram) – "anatomy scan"
A detailed look inside your belly to check for any problems with baby's growth or position. It can also check for certain birth defects. Done during weeks 18 to 22. See page 3 for more on ultrasounds.
Second trimester screening – "quad screen"
A blood test to check for common genetic defects. No risks. Done during weeks 15 to 22.
Glucose screening
A blood sugar test done to check for gestational diabetes. You drink a very sugary drink and then have a blood test an hour later. (If you do not pass, you will be offered a longer glucose test later.) Mild risk of stomach upset or dizziness. Done during weeks 24 to 28.

Diagnostic tests

If there is high risk or concern about genetic birth defects, you may choose to have an amniocentesis. Some people choose this instead of the first trimester CVS. It gives more information and has slightly less risk. Think back to the questions on page 102 to

What is gestational diabetes?

If you already have diabetes, your provider will talk with you about how to manage it while you are pregnant.

Gestational diabetes (GDM) only happens during pregnancy. It can cause severe problems for both mom and baby. Anyone can get GDM, but some people have more risk.

You should have a **glucose screen** each time you are pregnant. If your blood sugar is too high with the first test, you will go for a **glucose tolerance test**. If you do not pass that test, you will need to talk with your provider about what to do.

For most people, GDM can be managed with exercise and smart food choices. You may need to check your blood sugar and keep a food log. Some people need medicine. You and your baby may need to have your blood sugar checked during labor and after birth.

This type of diabetes goes away after birth.

help you decide. Are the answers you would get worth the small risks and side effects? Your provider can help you decide.

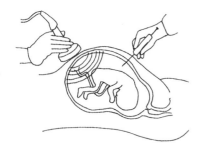

Amniocentesis (diagnostic)
A small amount of amniotic fluid is taken. The cells from the fluid are checked for genetic defects. The test uses an ultrasound to guide a very thin needle into the fluid near baby. Cramping is common, small risk of fluid leaking, bleeding, or infection. Very small risk of miscarriage.

Your body getting ready for labor

Braxton-Hicks contractions

Soon you will start to feel your uterus contracting. Your whole belly will get hard for a moment and then relax. These are called Braxton-Hicks contractions. They are normal and help your body get ready for real labor. They can feel strange, but they don't usually hurt. They start and stop a lot and don't get stronger. They will happen more as you get closer to your due date.

Preterm labor

When real labor starts before 37 weeks, it's called **preterm labor**. It is very serious. Often it can be stopped to give the baby more time to grow inside.

Warning signs – Preterm labor

Call your doctor or midwife right away if you have any of these signs:

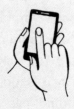

- ◆ Bleeding or pink or brown fluid coming from your vagina
- ◆ Loss of the mucus plug or clear fluid leaking from the vagina
- ◆ Contractions every 10 minutes or less, or cramps like those during your period
- ◆ Low back ache that may be steady or come and go
- ◆ Heavy feeling in your pelvis and vagina, like the baby is pushing down
- ◆ Unusual tightness or hardness of your belly
- ◆ A general feeling that something is wrong

Every day a baby stays inside your uterus helps him be better prepared for life outside. A baby born too early is more likely to have health problems. At 24 weeks (6 months), a baby may survive, but would need lots of special care.

Know the signs of preterm labor. These signs do not always mean preterm labor has started. However, it is best to call your health care provider right away.

Your doctor or midwife may want you to come in as soon as you can. Or she may ask you to lie on your left side and rest for an hour first. She may ask you to drink a few glasses of water or juice. Sometimes these things are enough to stop the contractions.

Some people are more likely to have preterm labor than others. Be sure to call your provider right away if you:

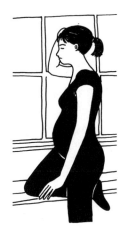

Watch out for mood changes. Hormones and lack of sleep can make these feelings much worse.

- have had a preterm baby before.

- are expecting more than one baby.

- are very stressed or afraid.

- have gum disease.

- have an infection or vaginal disease (uti, chlamydia, bacterial vaginosis).

- have been smoking or using alcohol or drugs.

Show these tips to your partner, if they haven't read the whole book!

Tips for partners

You are essential to your unborn baby's life, birth, and growth. Here are some things to do as you wait for birth.

Practical things

- Go to prenatal visits when you can.

- If you will be a birth partner, go to birth classes. Practice the coping skills together between classes.

- If you think you do not want to watch the birth, say so. You could help during labor and then leave the room when it's time to push.

- Brainstorm names for your baby.

Feelings

- Take time together. Do things now that will be harder after baby is born. Take a vacation. Get plenty of sleep.
- Hold your hand on your partner's tummy. Feel your baby move. Tell them what you will do when they're here.
- Pay attention to your moods and your partner's. Watch out for depression and anxiety.

Having sex

Some people love sex while pregnant and want to have a lot. In a healthy pregnancy, sex won't hurt baby. But, it is very important not to give your partner an STI right now.

Some may really want to but don't feel sexy or find sex awkward in these last months. Be kind and ask your partner what feels good. Try positions that don't push on your partner's belly, like having them on top.

Some people just don't feel sexual while pregnant. Their body is going through so much, it can be uncomfortable and tiring. If your partner avoids sex or seems to not enjoy it, talk to them. Remember, this isn't forever and there are other ways to be close.

Do not have sex if:

- your partner says no or avoids having sex.
- it seems like your partner has pain during sex or does not enjoy it.
- your partner is bleeding or leaking fluid from their vagina, or has any other signs of preterm labor. It's critical not to cause infection or strong contractions.

If you feel left out by your partner at this time, talk about it. They may be focused on your baby. Talking with each other about feelings is a good habit.

Monthly checkups

Questions to ask at your second trimester visits

- *Is my blood pressure normal?*
- *Can I keep exercising?*
- *I have not felt my baby move yet. Are they okay?*
- *If I have had a c-section before, must I have one again?*

Other questions you have:

1. _____

_____

2. _____

_____

Checkup notes

On this date, _____, I had my prenatal visit.

I am _____ weeks pregnant.

I weigh _____ pounds/kg now.

I have gained _____ pounds/kg since my last checkup.

I have gained _____ pounds/kg since I got pregnant.

My blood pressure is _____ /_____.

Things I learned today:

1. _____

_____

2. _____

_____

My next visit will be on

The _____ of _____, at _____:_____.

       (date)   **(month)**   **(time)**

Questions to ask at your next visit

- *Is my baby growing well?*
- *Is there any chance I could be having twins?*
- *Where can I find a good childbirth class?*
- *How long should I keep working?*
- *Is my blood pressure normal?*
- *What can I do about varicose veins?*

Other questions you have:

1. _____

_____

2. _____

_____

Checkup notes

On this date, _____, I had my prenatal visit.

I am _____ weeks pregnant.

I weigh _____ pounds/kg now.

I have gained _____ pounds/kg since my last checkup.

I have gained _____ pounds/kg since I got pregnant.

My blood pressure is _____/_____.

Things I learned today:

1. _____

_____

2. _____

_____

My next visit will be on

The _____ of _____, at ____:____.
    (date)   **(month)**   **(time)**

Questions to ask at next visit:

- *What can I do to get ready for breastfeeding?*
- *Am I likely to go into preterm labor?*
- *Why does my baby move a lot some days and not much on others?*
- *How do I know if I am getting enough exercise?*
- *Is my blood Rh negative?*
- *When will I have the test for gestational diabetes?*

Other questions you have:

1. _____

_____

2. _____

_____

Checkup notes

On this date, _____, I had my prenatal visit.

I am _____ weeks pregnant.

I weigh _____ pounds/kg now.

I have gained _____ pounds/kg since my last checkup.

I have gained _____ pounds/kg since I got pregnant.

My blood pressure is _____/_____.

Things I learned today:

1. _____

_____

2. _____

_____

Chapter 9

Your Third Trimester

Weeks 28 through 40 (until birth)

This is your last trimester! You have done a lot to help your baby be healthy. Your pregnancy is almost over. Are you eager to meet baby?

For months, your body has been getting ready for birth. Now is the time to read chapter 10. Go to a childbirth class.

Most important: Look back at page 120 in chapter 8 to be sure you know the signs of preterm labor. You may be getting tired of being pregnant, but your baby should stay safely inside your body until at least 39 weeks, if possible.

Look in this chapter for:

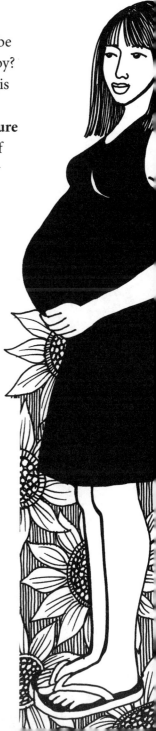

How your baby is growing

Weeks 28 through 31

This month, your baby will grow to be over ten inches long and weigh about 3 pounds. By the end of week 31, baby's:

- able to open their eyes and blink. They have eyelashes!
- lungs are formed, but are not ready to breathe air yet.
- hands can open and close.
- gaining weight quickly.

Weeks 32 through 35

Baby is getting more fat each week now. Their wrinkled skin is now plump and smooth. Baby will be about twelve inches long and weigh more than four pounds. By the end of week 35, baby's:

- bones are harder.
- arms and legs are smooth and chubby.
- startles and moves if you shine a bright light on your belly.
- fine lanugo falls off.
- finger and toe nails are longer.

Weeks 36 through 40

It's almost time! It is best for baby to stay in your body until 39 weeks. By then, baby may grow to be around twenty inches long and weigh between six to nine pounds. In these last weeks, baby's:

- lungs get ready to breathe air.
- gaining more fat to keep warm.
- crowded in there but you can still feel them roll and push.
- hopefully settling head-down to get ready for birth.

How your body is changing

Weeks 28 through 31

- You will gain a little more weight.
- You should still feel baby roll around. If they're moving a lot less, call your provider.

- Your feet and legs may swell. If your hands and face swell a lot, call your provider.
- It may be hard to keep your balance with your big belly. Be careful not to fall.
- You may feel very warm and have a hard time sleeping.
- You will probably feel Braxton-Hicks contractions.

Weeks 32 through 35

- You will gain a little more weight.
- Baby will push into your ribs.
- They will also push your stomach, lungs, and other organs aside. It may be hard to take a deep breath or eat a big meal.
- Your breasts may swell more and get sore. Colostrum may leak from your nipples.
- You may feel very warm. Wear light, loose clothes.
- You may leak urine when you sneeze, cough, or laugh.
- Your hip joints are getting looser and may ache. You may feel dizzy if you stand up suddenly. Try not to fall.

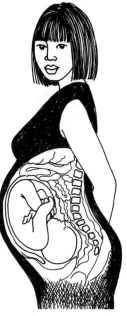

In the last three months, the growing baby pushes against your lungs, stomach, and intestines.

Weeks 36 through 40

- You will gain a little more weight.
- The baby will move down (drop) into your pelvis. They are getting into position for birth. You may feel like your uterus is pushing down on your cervix or bottom.
- Breathing and eating may be easier after this, but you may need to go pee more often. You also may get constipated more easily.
- Your cervix starts to get soft and thin before it opens.
- You may feel heavy and tired. Take time to rest.

Third trimester basics

Your to-do list

- Go to your prenatal checkups. You will have two in your eighth month and more in your last month.
- Go to your childbirth classes. Ask your birth partner to go with you. Practice the exercises that you learn.

"Just before my baby was born, I cleaned all the kitchen cabinets completely. I was amazed that I had the energy for it."

- Make your birth plan (later in this chapter). Talk it over with your provider at a checkup.
- Choose your baby's provider. (See chapter 5.)
- Learn about baby care. Your hospital, clinic, or community center may have classes. You won't have much time after baby is born.

Healthy habits – Keep 'em up!

- Continue to cook and eat healthy food like protein, veggies, and grains. And remember your prenatal vitamins.
- Drink at least eight tall glasses of water each day.
- Take a walk each day, even if it is a slow one.
- Stay away from alcohol, drugs, cigarettes, and smoke. Avoid people or places that make you feel unsafe.
- When driving, try to sit as far as possible from the steering wheel. If you are very short, this is really important.

Exercises to do now

As your belly gets bigger, make sure you don't give up on exercise. Look back at the exercises in chapters 3, 7, and 8. Make sure to do these two:

- Now it is more important than ever to keep your back strong, stand up straight, and pull in your belly. A growing baby will make your belly heavier. It will be easy to let it hang out.
- Stretching your hips will really help get you ready for birth. So practice now by sitting this way for a while every day. Try it on the floor or sitting on a firm chair without arms.

NO! YES!

Practice standing tall and pulling in your belly.

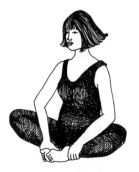

Sit on the floor to stretch your hips.

What to do if you can't sleep

It can be really hard to get good sleep in these months. As your baby gets bigger, it is harder to get comfortable. Your back and neck may ache. Your legs may cramp and your hips may hurt. It can be hard to breathe well and you may have heartburn. You probably need to get up often to go to the bathroom.

Try to be active every day. Even just a walk after dinner can help you sleep better. Try these tips for getting more rest:

- Nap when you can. Your body needs all the rest it can get right now.

- When settling down to rest, take deep breaths. Practice relaxation in the ways you learned in childbirth class.

- Lie on your left side. Put pillows under your back, belly, and neck. Add a big pillow between your knees.

- Avoid lying flat on your back for very long. This can be bad for you and baby.

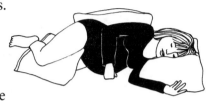

- Drink most of your water early in the day. Drink less later. This can help you get up less often to pee at night.

- Notice how you are feeling. Not sleeping could be a sign of depression or anxiety. (See chapter 16.)

Get comfortable—lie on your left side with pillows under your knee.

Baby's kicks and naps

Babies have quiet and active times each day. You probably will feel your baby move at least ten times in one to two hours. As you get closer to the birth, that may slow down. Baby doesn't have much room in there to move.

If you think baby has been moving a lot less for 24 hours, call your provider. They may want to check on baby.

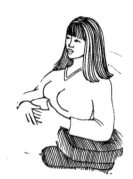

Feeling baby move

Prenatal testing

Testing in these last months depends on how your pregnancy is going and how your earlier tests went.

Routine tests

Non-stress test

A heart rate monitor is strapped onto your belly with a stretchy belt. This measures baby's heart beat for a time to look for signs of stress. No risk. Done during the last weeks before your due date. (It can be done sooner if there are concerns.)

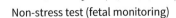

Non-stress test (fetal monitoring)

Group B Streptococcus (GBS)
A test to check for group B strep bacteria. GBS is harmless to you, but can very harmful to baby. If infected at birth, baby may suffer problems with their brain, lungs, or blood. To be safe, it is normal to test at the end of your pregnancy. A swab is used in your vagina and rectum. No risk.
Ultrasound
It is common to have an ultrasound if you get to 40 weeks with no signs of labor. This checks baby's position and how much fluid they have left around them. It is often done with a non-stress test.

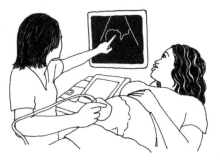

Special tests

If earlier tests do not go well, or there are other concerns, you may choose to have more tests. These can check baby's movement, breathing, blood flow, and even muscle tone. Most of these have no risk, but you can still ask questions before you decide.

Common worries

What if my blood pressure is high?

High blood pressure during pregnancy (also called **preeclampsia**, or **gestational hypertension**) can be very dangerous to you and your baby. If your blood pressure is high, you will need to take special care of yourself to prevent more serious problems. **Call your provider** if you have any warning signs. If it is after hours, call their emergency line.

Warning signs – High blood pressure

- Sudden weight gain (more than a pound in a day)
- Headache that will not go away
- Swollen hands and face
- Blurry vision or seeing spots
- Nausea and vomiting
- Trouble breathing

This could be an emergency. Call your doctor or midwife right away!

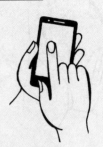

What if my baby's head isn't down?

Almost all babies are head-down and facing your back before birth. (This is called the **vertex position**.) This is the best position for birth. It is easiest for baby to move down and out head first. But your baby might be head-down, head-up (**breech**), or sideways (**transverse**). They may also be facing your back (**posterior**) or front (**anterior**). In these other positions, birth through the vagina would be hard. If baby doesn't turn before it's time for birth, a surgical birth may be the safest.

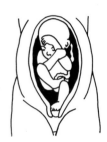

Baby in breech position with one leg down

How to help baby turn over

If your baby doesn't have their head down by 34 to 36 weeks, you may try to help them turn. Here are some gentle things you can do that might help to get them to flip.

- Try poses that open the pelvis and give space to baby to turn herself (breech tilt, sidelying, and **sifting**)
- Chiropractic care (Webster technique)
- Massage or craniosacral work (Maya massage or myofascial release)
- Sound, cold, relaxation (hypnosis, journaling, rest)
- Homeopathic remedy (moxibustion)

Breech tilt is a way to give baby space to turn naturally. Lie head down on a propped up ironing board.

These are not proven methods, but many people have found them helpful. Ask your provider if there's any reason why not to try any of these. See chapter 17 for resources to learn more.

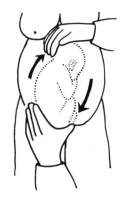

An external cephalic version (ECV) to change baby's position

If baby is not head-down as your due date gets closer, you can try gentle ways to get them to turn (see box on page 133 page). Or your doctor or midwife may try to get baby to turn by pushing on the outside of your uterus. This is called an **external cephalic version (ECV)**. They would use their hands on the outside of your belly to carefully push your baby into a new position. They'd watch baby's heart rate while pushing to make sure it doesn't cause too much stress. It doesn't feel good, but it can help you avoid surgery.

If your provider doesn't turn your baby or other measures don't work, they would likely say that a c-section is safest. See chapter 10 to learn more.

Your body getting ready for labor

Pre-labor contractions

The mild Braxton-Hicks contractions you may have been feeling will get stronger closer to the birth. Sometimes these contractions feel so strong that you might think they are the real thing. They may be called "false labor." If you have given birth before, Braxton-Hicks contractions may feel stronger this time.

Look back at the ways to tell if you're having pre-term labor contractions (chapter 8). If contractions start to come regularly and get stronger, they may be real labor. (Learn more of the signs of real labor in chapter 10.)

Your last prenatal visits

Your provider will want check you more often in the last few weeks of pregnancy. They may check:

 • how far down baby has moved.
 • baby's position.
 • how much the cervix has changed.

Your cervix starts to thin (efface) and open (dilate) in the last month. You may not feel this happening. Usually, it will change faster when you go into active labor.

The thick mucus plug from your cervix may come out with a little blood (called **bloody show**).

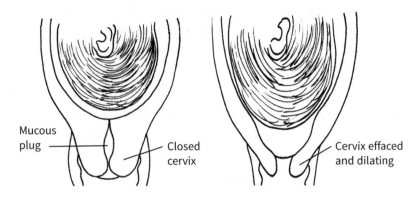

Mucous plug

Closed cervix

Cervix effaced and dilating

How your cervix opens

Effacement is the thinning of the neck of the cervix. **Dilation** is the opening of the hole. Both things happen as the baby's body presses down on the cervix.

Last steps to get your body ready

You can do many things to get yourself ready for labor.

Stay active. Continue the exercises and stretches from chapters 3 and 8 as long as they are comfortable. Remember that squats, kegels, and massage all help you get ready for pushing. Practice tightening and relaxing.

Practice relaxing during contractions. Use your Braxton-Hicks contractions to practice what you have learned about relaxing. As your belly gets hard, try the ways of breathing that you learned in birth classes.

Having sex can help you get ready for labor, too. If you want to and your provider does not say not to, you can have sex until your water breaks. You may feel contractions if you have an orgasm. Semen can also help thin the cervix. And the hormones and good feelings from sex can help you relax. See chapter 8 for more.

Get comfortable. Standing up straight, lying on your left side, and using lots of pillows will help you in these last months. Look at the tips for getting rest earlier in this chapter. Go back to chapter 8 for more tips on staying comfortable.

Be patient.

Most babies know when it's time to be born. The closer to 40 weeks baby is born, the healthier they are likely to be. Baby's brain and lungs are still developing in the last few weeks.

Once you reach 37 weeks (early term), you don't need to worry if labor starts on its own. But if labor starts before that, your provider may try to stop it so baby can stay in longer. You may need to be on bed rest until baby is born. Some babies are born early no matter what you do. It doesn't mean you did anything wrong. You took great care of baby all those months they were inside you.

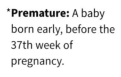

Premature: A baby born early, before the 37th week of pregnancy.

Premature* babies (**preemies**) often need to stay in the hospital for a time. They may need extra care while they catch up on the growing they would have done inside in those last weeks. See chapters 10 and 11 to learn more.

Read chapter 10

Know as much as you can about birth before it starts. You won't want to try to learn as you go, although your nurses, doctor, or midwife will be able to help you.

Know signs of labor starting

Put a bookmark in page 152 where it lists many of the signs of labor.

Talk to your provider about what to do when you think labor is starting. You might ask:

- *How do I know I'm really in labor?*
- *When do I call you?*
- *When do I come in?*

Give your other kids extra attention now

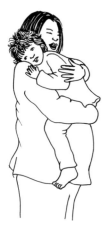

Make sure your older kids know you will have plenty of love for all of them.

Let your older kids know that you will have the baby soon. Tell them what the plan is—when you may leave, who will stay with them, and when you will be back. Think of something special they can do, either for their own fun or to welcome baby. Let them know when they will be able to see you and meet baby.

Baby can hear all of the sounds around you. It may feel silly at first, but urge your kids to talk to baby before birth. That way, baby will know their voices and may react to them when they finally meet.

If you are planning a home birth, think about if you want your other kids there with you. You would need to tell them what to expect. The sights and sounds of labor and delivery could be scary. If they are old enough to understand, ask them if they want to be there. Talk with your midwife about how to prepare them.

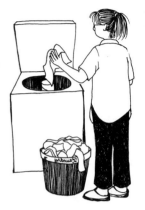

It's best to have someone you trust come over to care for them even if they say they want to be with you. That way, they could change their minds, go out, have food, and play while you and your partner are busy.

Get the practical things done

☐ Register at the hospital or birth center ahead of time. This will make everything easier when you arrive in labor.

Ask relatives and friends to help around the house.

☐ Pack your bag. (See chapter 10 for a list of things to take along.)

☐ Plan how to get to the hospital. Who will drive you? You might want to ask more than one person in case one is busy. Does that person know how to get there?

☐ Check with friends who have said they would help after you come home. Make sure they can do it.

☐ Choose baby's doctor or nurse. Look back at chapter 5 for tips on making this big decision.

Things to have ready at home

☐ Some cooked meals in the freezer

☐ Menstrual pads (not tampons)

☐ Diapers and other baby supplies

☐ Mild laundry soap for baby's clothes

Write down your birth plan

A birth plan is a list or letter about how you want your labor and birth to go. It's a tool to talk with your provider about what kind of care you want. If you give birth in a hospital, it helps the nurses, doctors, and midwives know your goals. It will also help you and your support person(s) keep track of the decisions you've made.

What to include

Make your birth plan after you have learned all about labor and birth. Talk to your childbirth class leader about what to put in it. Ask your doctor, midwife, or nurse, too. Providers are more likely to read it if it fits on one page, so think about what's most important to you.

No matter what kind of birth you end up having, you will have choices to make. Think about your perfect birth. What makes it perfect for you and for baby?

Now, think about some of the tricky things that could come up during labor and birth. What do you feel strongly about? Write those down, too. It's very hard to think clearly in labor, so having things written down is helpful.

What else?

If you are planning a home birth or birth center birth, it's a good idea to make a "plan B" birth plan for in case you end up in the hospital. Ask your provider what things you should include. (Go back to chapter 5 to review what is different in the hospital.)

Write down any choices you've made about how you want your baby to be cared for right after birth, too.

Be real with your goals

It's important to think about your goals before you're in labor. It helps everyone around you support you and your baby. When you talk to your providers, ask them what they think of your plan. Sometimes hospital rules get in the way of some goals. Sometimes you and your provider may feel very differently about something. A birth plan is also a way to let them know what you feel strongly about, are scared of, and are excited about. Some things can be argued, but your feelings can't. This can help your partner or care team work with you.

What do you do with the plan?

Ask to have it put in your chart. Bring a few copies with you to your birth. If in the hospital, ask the nurse to post it by the door or on the front of your chart.

My Birth Plan

These are my wishes. I know I can change my mind at any time. I also know the things I want may not happen if problems come up.

Name: _____

- My birth partner/support team for labor: _____
- I want to be able to walk around during labor. Yes ___ No ___
- I want to have medication as early as possible. Yes ___ No ___
- I want no pain medication. Yes ___ No ___
- If I need medication, I'd like this kind: _____
- How will I decide I need them? _____
- I would like to try these positions during labor: (circle) standing, sitting, squatting, other _____ .
- I do not want an episiotomy if possible. Please use other methods to avoid tearing or cutting. Yes ___ No ___
- I would like _____ to cut the cord.
- I want to breastfeed my baby right away. Yes ___ No ___

   I would like my baby to get breastmilk only until we go home. Yes ___ No ___
- I want my baby to stay in my room all the time. Yes ___ No ___
- In case of a c-section, I would like to to watch or have the doctor tell me what is happening. Yes ___ No ___ .
- My birth partner wants to be with me during the c-section. Yes ___ No ___
- If I have a baby boy, I want them to be circumcised. Yes ___ No ___
- I want medicine to be used to reduce the baby's pain. Yes ___ No ___
- I and my partner want to be present at the circumcision. Yes ___ No ___
- The circumcision will be a religious ceremony. Yes ___ No ___
- Other things I want my caregivers to know to know:

   _____

   _____

   _____

   _____

   _____

Remember that each labor and birth is different. Things may not go the way you put in your birth plan. Or, you may change your mind about something. You birth plan is just your goals. If things change, ask questions until you feel okay about what's happening. Don't be afraid to ask your providers to explain things. If it is emergency, they won't let your questions keep them from helping you or your baby.

Tips for partners

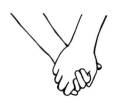

- Be ready. Know the signs of labor. Know when to call the doctor, midwife, or nurse. Know when to go to the hospital or birth center, and how to get there.

- Watch out for the warning signs of high blood pressure (see page 133) and call right away if you are concerned.

- Practice what you learned to help your partner relax during labor.

- Talk about the birth plan. Be sure you know what your partner wants and doesn't want so you can support them when it's time.

- Be patient. Your partner may be very tired and uncomfortable in these last weeks. Help them stay relaxed as you both wait for baby.

Monthly checkups

Month 7

Questions to ask at my seven-month checkup

- *How long should I plan to keep working?*
- *Am I likely to go into labor early (preterm labor)?*
- *Do I have inverted nipples?*
- *I eat lots of vegetables, fruit, and grains but still get constipated. What else can I do?*
- *Should I start counting how often my baby moves?*
- *If you are expecting twins: Is there anything special I should know to prevent preterm labor?*

Other questions I have:

1. _____

   _____

   _____

2. _____

   _____

   _____

3. _____

   _____

   _____

Your seven-month checkup notes

Today, _____, I had my seven-month appointment.

I am _____ weeks pregnant. I weigh _____ pounds/kg.

I have gained _____ pounds/kg since my last checkup.

My blood pressure is _____/_____ (see below).

Things I learned today

1. _____

_____

2. _____

_____

3. _____

_____

My next checkup will be on

The _____ of _____, at _____:_____.
      (date)   (month)   (time)

Questions to ask at your next checkup

- *Is my baby growing well?*
- *Can my partner and I still have sex and what positions are best at this time?*
- *Is my baby head down or head up?*
- *How is my blood pressure?*
- *What kind of exercise should I do now?*
- *How do I register at the hospital or birth center before I go into labor?*

Other questions I have:

1. _____

_____

_____

2. _____

_____

_____

3. _____

_____

_____

My eight-month checkup #1 notes

On this date, _____, I had my first eight-month appointment.

I am _____ weeks pregnant. I weigh _____ pounds/kg.

I have gained _____ pounds/kg since my last checkup.

My blood pressure is _____/_____.

My baby's position: _____.

Things I learned today:

1. _____

   _____

2. _____

   _____

3. _____

   _____

My doctor or nurse-midwife wants me to call when I have these signs of labor:

1. _____

   _____

2. _____

   _____

3. _____

   _____

4. _____

   _____

My next checkup will be on

The _____ of _____, at ____:____.
   (date)   (month)   (time)

My eight-month checkup #2 notes

On this date, _____, I had my second eight-month appointment.

I am _____ weeks pregnant. I weigh _____ pounds/kg now.

I have gained _____ pounds/kg since my last checkup.

I have gained _____ pounds/kg since I got pregnant.

My blood pressure is _____/_____.

Things I learned today:

1. _____

_____

2. _____

_____

My next checkup will be on

The _____ of _____, at ____:_____.
    (date)   (month)   (time)

Questions to ask at your nine-month checkups

- *How will I know if my contractions are real labor? When should I call you?*
- *What positions (sitting, squatting, or lying down) do you think work best during labor?*
- *If I need pain medication, what kinds would you advise? What side effects would they have for my baby and me?*
- *Who can help me with breastfeeding?*
- *Do I need a group B strep test?*

Other questions I have:

1. _____

_____

2. _____

_____

Use the last page of this chapter to write things you want to remember about this important time.

My nine-month checkup #1 notes

On this date, _____, I had my second eight-month appointment.

I weigh _____ pounds/kg now.

I have gained _____ pounds/kg since my last checkup.

My blood pressure is _____/_____.

My baby has dropped? Yes ___ No ___

I am _____ percent effaced and _____ centimeters dilated. (This may not be measured at every checkup this month.)

My baby's position is head down ___ or bottom down ___.

Things I learned today:

1. _____

_____

2. _____

_____

3. _____

_____

My next checkup will be on

The _____ of _____, at ____:____.
    (date)   (month)   (time)

(Notes pages for the next few weekly visits are at the end of this chapter.)

My nine-month checkup #2 notes

Date _____

I weigh _____ pounds/kg now.

I have gained _____ pounds/kg since I got pregnant.

My blood pressure is _____/_____.

I am _____ percent effaced and _____ centimeters dilated (if measured).

Things I learned today:

1. _____

_____

2. _____

_____

My next checkup will be on

The _____ of _____, at _____:_____.
    (date)   **(month)**   **(time)**

My nine-month checkup #3 notes

Date _____ I weigh _____ pounds/kg now.

I am _____ percent effaced and _____ centimeters dilated (if measured).

Things I learned today

1. _____

_____

2. _____

_____

My next checkup will be on

The _____ of _____, at _____:_____.
    (date)   **(month)**   **(time)**

My nine-month checkup #4 notes

Date _____ I weigh _____ pounds/kg now.

My blood pressure is _____/_____.

I am _____ percent effaced and _____ centimeters dilated (if measured).

Things I learned today:

1. _____

   _____

2. _____

   _____

3. _____

   _____

How I am feeling now:

_____

_____

_____

_____

_____

_____

_____

   You can keep notes on what happened during labor and delivery at the end of chapter 10.

The big day is almost here!

Whether your pregnancy has been easy or not, you know it will end soon. You will soon have a new child to love. You have already started to be a parent by taking care of your unborn baby.
What names are you thinking of giving your baby?

_____

_____

_____

How do you feel now?

___ Excited ___ Scared ___ Happy ___ Depressed
___ A little bit of all of these

Other feelings?

_____

_____

_____

What are your special hopes?

_____

_____

_____

Do you have new concerns now?

_____

_____

_____

Share how you feel with your partner or with a close friend.

_____

_____

_____

Chapter 10

Your Baby's Birth

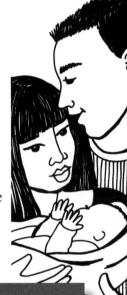

By now, you probably feel very tired of being pregnant and ready to move on to parenthood. As you wait for your baby's birth, you likely feel both excited and worried.

Giving birth is a natural and amazing thing. It may seem strange and intense, but your body will know what to do. Learning what to expect can help you feel ready and make birth less scary.

This chapter will tell you all about normal birth—what birth is like when it happens smoothly all on its own. It also describes some common medical ways of helping if you or baby need help along the way.

Look in this chapter for:

Be ready ahead of time

Learning all there is to know about labor and birth can be a lot to take in. Reading this chapter before your last month of pregnancy will help you plan ahead.

   If you have not had a chance to take a birth class, tell your provider. They can help make sure you know what to expect and get your questions answered. Look at the birth resources in chapter 17. There are great videos and short overviews that can help you feel prepared.

Your birth plan

Remember the birth plan in chapter 9? If you haven't done it, do it now. Reading this chapter will help you decide about your wishes. Give the plan to your provider and make sure your birth partner has a copy.

Information for the hospital or birth center
Fill this out before labor begins:

Your blood type (ask your provider) _____

Any problems with your pregnancy? (diabetes, high blood pressure, etc.) _____

_____

Your doctor or midwife_____

Phone # _____ 24-hour phone # _____

Baby's doctor or nurse _____

Phone # _____ 24-hour phone # _____

Insurance company or plan _____

Your policy # _____

Your birth partner (name and phone #)

_____

Do you have a birth plan? no __ yes __ (If yes, where is it?)

_____

Your contacts in an emergency: (names and phone numbers)

_____

_____

What should I take with me?

Pack most of these things ahead of time. Check off each thing as you pack it.

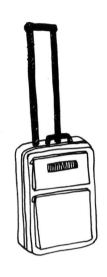

____ Your ID and insurance card.

____ Your birth plan.

____ This book.

____ A watch with a second hand or a smart phone with a timer for timing contractions.

____ A pen and paper for notes.

____ A way to play your favorite music. Soft, quiet music can help you relax during labor.

____ Your phone and charger.

____ A camera with full battery (if your phone is not a good option).

____ Sugar-free candy to keep your mouth moist.

____ Clothes or a nightgown to wear if you don't want to use a hospital gown. Take a short robe or sweater that opens in front, slippers, and warm socks.

____ Hairbrush, hair ties, toothbrush, and toothpaste. Prescription medicines.

____ Other things that may help you feel fresh, like face wash, deodorant, lotion, or makeup.

____ Money for your birth partner(s) to buy coffee and food.

____ Snacks to help keep you both going. Dried fruit, nut butter, and cheese or yogurt can give you energy.

____ A nursing bra.

____ Stretchy or loose clothes to wear home.

____ Clothes for baby to wear home: an outfit with legs, socks, and a hat. (Gowns don't let the car-seat harness fit safely.)

____ A few thin baby blankets and one thick one.

____ Car seat for the ride home. You and your baby must ride buckled up, even in a taxi. If you do not have a car seat, ask if the hospital sells low-cost seats.

How birth happens on its own

No one can say for sure when your labor will start, but you can be sure it will happen soon. Some people have clear signs before it begins. Others do not.

In the last few weeks before the birth, your baby drops (moves down) between the pelvic bones. You may see your belly is lower. Your cervix softens, thins, and starts to opens. (See pictures, chapter 9, page 135.) Now your real contractions will begin.

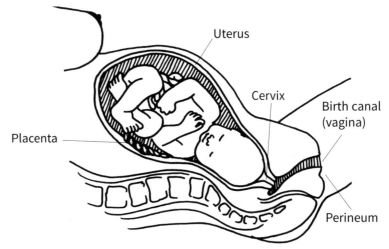

Uterus

Cervix

Birth canal
(vagina)

Placenta

Perineum

Baby in the uterus—parts to know

Labor usually starts any time from two weeks before your due date to two weeks after. Labor may last a few hours or more than a day. Labor often will take longer the first time than with second or third babies.

Try to be patient. A baby's body needs at least 39 weeks in the uterus. Their brain, lungs, and liver are still growing. Babies born too soon do not have fat to stay warm. They also may not be able to see or hear as well.

Is labor starting?

There are many signs of labor. You may not have all of them. Ask your doctor or midwife what else to watch for.

- ◆ A glob of thick mucus (called the **mucus plug**) with a little bright red blood that comes out of your vagina.

When to call your doctor or midwife

Ask your provider when to call. Write it here:

_____

_____

When in doubt, call if:

- ◆ Your bag of waters breaks.
- ◆ Your contractions have been 5 to 10 minutes apart for at least an hour.
- ◆ You cannot walk or talk during contractions.

Tell your provider as much as you can about what is going on. If you can't talk, ask your partner to talk for you.

- ◆ Clear* fluid that gushes or leaks from your vagina. This is the bag of waters (amniotic sac) breaking. This may happen before or after contractions start.
- ◆ Low back pain that will not go away or low belly cramps (like when you have your period). You may even feel a rhythm.
- ◆ Very soft bowel movements (or diarrhea).
- ◆ Contractions that get stronger, last longer, and come closer and closer together.

*If your waters break but it is not clear, be sure to tell your provider. If there is poop in the fluid, they will make sure baby's lungs sound clear after birth.

Call any time, day or night. It is better to call early than to wait too long. You may be asked to stay at home for a while, or to take a walk close by. If your water has broken, your provider will likely want to see you within a few hours.

Ask when you should go to the hospital or birth center. If you are planning a home birth, ask when they will come over.

Is it real labor?

It can be hard to tell if your contractions are real. You've felt contractions on and off in the last months. Try these things:

- ◆ Lie down and rest for a while.
- ◆ Get up and walk around.
- ◆ Drink a big glass of water and have a small snack.

If doing these things make the contractions stop or get weaker or slower, you're probably not really in labor. Real labor contractions don't stop coming once they start.

Time your contractions (see pages 158 on how to time). Early contractions are about a half-minute long and come about every 15 to 30 minutes.

If you are not sure, call your doctor or midwife. They will not mind being called at any time. Sometimes the only way to know if true labor has started is to be checked by your provider. They can feel where baby is and how much your cervix has changed.

STAGE 1: Labor

During pregnancy, the uterus has grown into the largest, strongest muscle in your body. When labor starts, it contracts without any help from you. This can feel very strange at first.

Your job is to help the uterus by letting it do its work. Relax as much as you can during contractions and rest in between. Move around, like walking or trying different positions. Stay upright by standing, sitting, squatting, or kneeling. Just lying down in bed can slow labor.

What's going on during labor

Your body is working hard to do two important jobs:

+ Get your cervix ready. It must get thin (efface) and open up wide (dilate). These things all make it easier for baby to pass through.

+ Get baby ready. Baby needs to move down low into your pelvis for birth. The more open your cervix is, the lower baby can get. This can feel like your belly drops down and is called "lightening."

The basic stages of labor

1st Stage: Labor (Opening of the cervix)

The cervix opens (dilates) and thins (effaces) to let the baby through. Contractions become stronger and faster as the uterus pushes baby down into the cervix. This is the longest stage of childbirth.

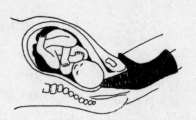

2nd Stage: Birth of your baby (Delivery)

With your help, the uterus contractions push baby through the open cervix, into the vagina. The vagina and perineum stretch wide open and the baby comes out.

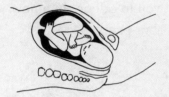
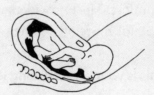
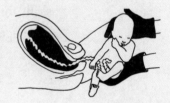

In the second stage, the baby is first pushed all the way down the birth canal.

Next, the baby's head comes out the vagina.

Last, the baby's body comes out.

3rd Stage: Delivery of the placenta

The placenta comes off the wall of the uterus. The uterus contracts to push it out through the vagina. This stage is much less painful. Baby may be put on your chest during this stage and for recovery.

4th Stage: Recovery

The uterus starts to shrink while you rest and relax. This is a good time to breastfeed and talk to your baby. Baby will be checked and warmed up. All this can be done while baby is on your chest. You will get stitches if you have a tear or cut in your perineum.

Labor is often talked about in 2 parts. How long each part lasts is different for everyone. Your provider may have tips for how to tell the difference or when to call them or go in.

Early labor

"I baked a birthday cake to help the time go by! It was fun!"

Contractions are short and not very often. **Your cervix opens to 6 cm.** This is the longest part of labor and can last many hours, or even days. Most people spend early labor at home. This is a great time to watch a movie, relax with friends, or even go for a walk.

Active labor

Contractions are longer (45–60 seconds), stronger, and closer together (every 3–4 minutes). **Your cervix opens to 10 cm.** Most people can't ignore these contractions and need to use coping skills for comfort. Most providers want you to call or go in now. See page 158 for more on coping with labor pain.

This is your cervix during labor

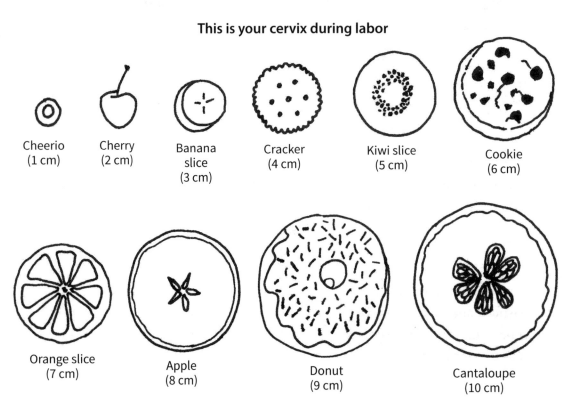

Cheerio
(1 cm)

Cherry
(2 cm)

Banana
slice
(3 cm)

Cracker
(4 cm)

Kiwi slice
(5 cm)

Cookie
(6 cm)

Orange slice
(7 cm)

Apple
(8 cm)

Donut
(9 cm)

Cantaloupe
(10 cm)

The opening of your cervix will stretch from 1 cm to 10 cm.
That's like going from a Cheerio to a cantaloupe!

More about early labor

Early labor can take a few hours or a few days. You will be more comfortable at home at this time. There is no need to be in the hospital or birth center until you are in active labor. Getting to the hospital early does not help your baby come quicker and you may be sent home.

Bookmark page 152 for signs of labor and when to call your doctor or midwife. Also, call if you or the baby suddenly feel different or if you have questions.

While you are in early labor, you can do some normal things, like cook, take a walk, watch a movie, and visit with friends. Eat lightly and drink water or juice. Try to relax and take naps, but don't just lie down the whole time. Sitting up, standing, and walking help the baby move down into the birth canal. Let gravity help pull baby down.

During a contraction, try the breathing and relaxation exercises you have learned. Have your partner time your contractions so you know when to call your provider.

If you see any warning signs of high blood pressure, call right away. See page 133.

Active labor – When things get harder

Once you are checked in to the hospital, a labor and delivery nurse will help you know what to do. If you go to a birth center or are at home, your midwife will help guide you. These nurses and midwives have helped many families in labor. They will have a lot of tips for you and your partner or birth team. Their advice about positions, what to do, and how to breathe can be very helpful. If you have a doctor, they will likely check in on you from time to time. They'll likely come back and stay when you start to push. Until then, nurses will be with you to help.

Tips for partners – Keep track of contractions

Knowing how long, strong, and far apart your contractions are is an important role for a birth partner. This will tell both of you and your provider how labor is going. Use a timer or a watch with a second hand to time contractions. Put the information into the form in the box on the next page.

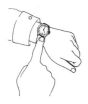

How to time contractions

Write the exact time when each contraction starts and stops. Figure out how long they last and how far apart they are (from start time to start time).

Note other things that happen, such as the bag of waters breaking.

Start time	Stop time	How long was it?	How far apart?*	Other Signs
_____	_____	_____	_____	_____
_____	_____	_____	_____	_____
_____	_____	_____	_____	_____
_____	_____	_____	_____	_____
_____	_____	_____	_____	_____
_____	_____	_____	_____	_____

(Use another piece of paper to continue your notes.)

*Count how many minutes pass from the start of one contraction to the start of the next one.

Comfort in labor

Staying calm and relaxed helps labor go more smoothly and hurt less. Make sure the nurses or your midwife have your birth plan.

Drink water or juice or suck on ice chips to stay hydrated. Go to the bathroom as you need to. Many people find sitting on the toilet very comfortable in labor.

It will be easier to relax in a quiet, peaceful room. Play music that you like. Post a "quiet" sign on the door or ask people to wait outside if you feel the need.

Most people do not go through labor lying down. Moving around and being upright can be more comfortable and help labor move along.

Some positions to try:

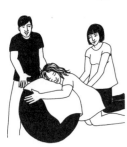

Two comfortable positions

- ◆ Walk or slow-dance with your partner.
- ◆ Stand and lean back or forward into your partner.
- ◆ Rest on your hands and knees.
- ◆ Fold your arms on a birth ball while kneeling.
- ◆ Squat and lean back or forward into your partner.

If active labor goes on for a long time, gets too painful for you, or you start to feel too tired to go on, you may want to ask for some pain medicine.

Coping with pain

Pain will be a natural part of your baby's birth. You do not need to be scared. It comes from the work your body is doing.

Most labor pain comes from the squeezing of the uterus, the widening of the birth canal and pelvis, the stretching of the perineum. Stress, pain, and contractions all make the body release natural pain control (endorphins). This can be very powerful.

Labor pain often starts as a dull back ache or cramps that come and go. The cramping gets much stronger as contractions come closer together and last longer. As you start to push, the stretching of your pelvis, vagina, and perineum will hurt. Once baby is out, almost all of the pain is gone right away. Then, your baby can help distract you from the rest.

Giving birth without drugs can make you feel very good and very strong. If your labor is going well, you may only need some relaxation and comfort methods to get you through it.

Tips for having less pain

- Have a birth partner and/or a doula to support, comfort, and encourage you.
- Use breathing and massage methods to relax.
- Change positions—sit up, squat, kneel, get on hands and knees, sit on a birth ball, rock in a rocker.
- Squeeze a hairbrush or comb in your hand to distract from the pain.
- Walk slowly as your partner holds you.
- Sit in a shower or soak in a warm (not hot) tub—after you are at least 6 cm dilated.
- Focus on the important job you are doing and know it won't last much longer.

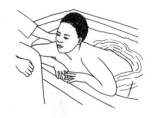

Help for back pain

Contractions can make your back tired and sore. This pain can be very strong if baby is facing your front. (Most babies face the back during labor.) When baby faces front, their head pushes hard on your bones, which can hurt a lot. Try the comfort methods above. Here are other things that can help:

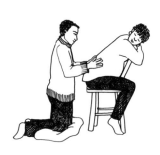

- ◆ Have your partner push firmly on your low back.
- ◆ Put a heat pad or cold pack on your low back.
- ◆ Let your partner massage your back and hips.
- ◆ Lean forward against your partner, a table or bed, or on a birth ball. Or rest your head on a pillow while you kneel on a bed or the ground. These poses take the strain off of your back and let let your belly just hang.

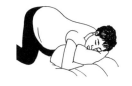

- ◆ Lie on your side if you get in bed. Try and rest.
- ◆ Get in the shower and have your partner spray the water on your low back. Close your eyes and relax.

When you need more help – Pain medicine

Coping with pain can make you very tired. If labor goes on very long, you may need more help for the pain. Asking for help doesn't mean you did anything wrong.

There are a few types of medicine that can help. Some help you relax and not be so afraid of labor pain. Some give you a break from the pain so you can rest and get your strength back. Others numb your body so you don't feel the pain. **See page 166 to learn more.**

Tips for partners – During active labor

Your biggest job is to help your partner relax during contractions and stay comfortable. You could:

- ◆ Keep timing the contractions.
- ◆ Help them change positions, offer back or foot rubs.
- ◆ Support them while they walk around or use the bathroom.
- ◆ Offer ice chips or foods that are okay to have.
- ◆ Help with the relaxation methods you both learned in class.

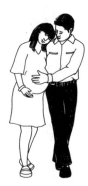

You are your partner's protector during labor. All focus should be on their comfort and needs.

- ◆ Keep the room quiet or play sounds or music they choose; ask staff or visitors to go out of the room to talk.

- Make sure the nurses or midwife have the birth plan. If you notice the plan isn't being followed, ask why.

- Speak up if you think your partner is having problems. Ask the nurse or midwife to make sure things are okay.

- Keep yourself strong by eating, drinking, and taking breaks when you need to.

From labor to birth: Transition

The end of labor is called transition. When your cervix is ready, your labor may seem to pause for a moment. Then, contractions come hard and fast. You may feel very tired and not be able to talk much or focus. You may feel shaky or like you need to vomit. This can be the hardest part, but it is also very short. And, it means baby is coming soon!

You may start to feel a strong urge to push. This may feel like pressure in your bottom or the need to lean over your belly. It is best to let your provider check your cervix before you push. If it's not all the way open, pushing can lead to problems.* Once your cervix is ready, it's baby time!

*If your provider says not to push, try slow, deep breaths and gentle swaying. Very gentle massage or brushing fingers over your back, belly, or legs may help.

STAGE 2: The birth of your baby!

When it's time to push, try to focus on your breathing. Your midwife or nurse can help guide you to take a few quick breaths with each push. Try not to hold your breath. Each push helps stretch your vagina and move baby down the birth canal. In between contractions, try to rest and take slow, deep breaths.

This stage can take a long time. After a while, your provider will check how far down baby has come. Help baby along by spending some time walking, sitting, or squatting. These positions allow gravity to help.

When it is time to push, try to take a few quick breaths as you push through each contraction. Rest in between, taking deep breaths. At times, your provider may ask you *not* to push. This lets them check on baby's cord or position. This also gives time for the perineum to stretch. Blowing out lots of short breaths in a row or low moaning can help you to not push.

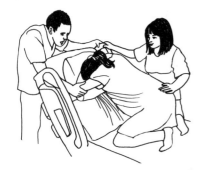 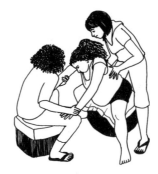 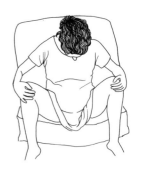

A few good pushing poses

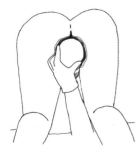

***Crowning** is when you can see the top of baby's head coming out.

When the baby's head is all the way down in your vagina, your provider can see it. Your perineum must stretch wide enough for it. The skin may burn or sting.

Ways your provider can help baby come through the perineum more easily include:

- slowing down delivery a little by holding their hand on baby's head.
- using a warm cloth or gentle massage to help avoid tearing.
- making a cut in the perineum to widen the opening (an episiotomy). (See page 167–168.)

Even if the opening is wide enough, sometimes a baby's head won't come out as it should. The provider may use forceps or a vacuum extractor to keep baby from slipping back in between pushes. This will guide baby's head out. See page 168 to learn more about these tools.

Once your baby's head and shoulders are out, the rest of their body slips out quickly. You will feel great relief and have much less pain.

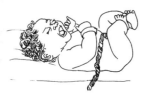

When baby first comes out, they may be very still and quiet. The doctor or midwife may clear the nose and mouth to help baby take their first breath. Baby will likely cry as their lungs fill with air for the first time.

If you ask, your provider will likely put baby right on your chest or belly. It is good for you and baby to be skin to skin for the first hour or so. Finally, you can hold the baby you worked so hard for!

Cutting the cord

After birth, your provider will clamp and cut the cord. Cutting the cord does not hurt you or your baby. Your partner may want to cut the cord.

You may want to ask your provider to wait until the cord stops pulsing to clamp the cord. This lets more of baby's blood move from the placenta into their body. This can help give baby a healthy start.

Tips for partners – During baby's birth

- Help your partner get into positions to help baby come out.
- Use a cool cloth to wipe their forehead.
- Believe in your partner and the hard work they're doing. Offer kind words and stay calm.
- Remind your partner it's almost time to meet baby. Tell them when baby's head starts to show.
- Stay calm and quiet, so they can focus and rest, and so they can hear their provider.
- If you want to and your partner agrees, ask to cut the cord. It won't hurt and it's something special you can do.

STAGE 3: Delivery of the placenta

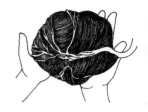

In a few more minutes, the placenta will come off the wall of your uterus. Contractions will continue to push it out, but they will be much more gentle. You may not even feel them. Or your provider may ask you to push a few more times.

Your provider will check to make sure all of it has come out. Your nurse or midwife may rub your belly firmly to help your tired uterus. You may get some medicine to help it stop bleeding.

Tips for partners – After baby is out

- Ask the nurse to bring a warm blanket, and get a snack and drink for your partner.
- Ask them not to give baby a bath yet so you can spend time together first.

STAGE 4: Beginning of recovery

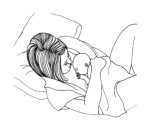

You did it! Now your nurse or midwife will help you get cleaned up and comfortable.

If you had an episiotomy or tear, your doctor or midwife will stitch it up. This can take a few minutes. They will numb the area so you don't feel it.

Now you can relax. You can cuddle and nurse your baby. Drink some water or juice, eat, and rest.

Your uterus should start shrinking right away. You may feel more contractions. Your nurse or midwife will feel your belly and may massage your uterus to help it shrink down. You may be able to feel it yourself. Reach down and press on your lower belly. Your uterus should feel hard and be about the size of a grapefruit.

This is a great time to try nursing. New babies are usually awake and eager to feed in the first hour after birth. Your baby will know the smell of your breast milk. It smells like the amniotic fluid they've been in. If baby doesn't want to nurse, let them lie on your chest with their face on your breast.

You will have bleeding from your vagina for at least a few weeks. You will need to wear large pads or postpartum underwear. (No tampons or cups!)

Tips for partners – Help with care

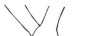

- Enjoy this time with your partner and new baby.
- Help with breastfeeding.
- Try kangaroo care (skin to skin) when baby isn't nursing. Open your shirt and cuddle baby on your bare chest. Put a warm blanket over both of you.
- Offer to help your partner freshen up. Pulling their hair back or using a warm face cloth can feel good.

Other things you may need to know

Sometimes your body or baby need a bit more help during labor or birth. "Interventions" are things your provider can do to help things along safely. Learn about them before you go into labor. If your provider suggests one of these things, it is good to know a bit about it. This helps you make choices that feel right to you.

Ask your provider:

- *How will this help me?*
- *How soon do we have to decide?*
- *What are the benefits and risks?*
- *Are there any other ways that might be less risky?*

You can always say you want to know more before giving consent (saying that it's okay). But, if there is a true emergency, your provider will say so and do what is needed.

Induction – Helping labor start

Labor can be started (induced) using drugs or other ways to get the cervix to open and contractions to start. It is usually best to wait for your body to start labor naturally. This is why most providers do not want to start labor early "just to get it over with."

But, there are some important medical reasons to try to start labor. A common reason is if a baby is late. Late means two weeks after their due date (42 weeks). Until then, most babies are safest staying in the belly. After 42 weeks, there is more risk of problems for both you and baby.

If baby is overdue, your doctor or midwife will likely check your cervix often to see if it is opening. To get labor started they might suggest:

- things to try at home, like going for walks, climbing stairs, having sex, or playing with your nipples.
- a membrane sweep: a provider slides a gloved finger into the uterus and moves the bag of waters away from the uterine wall.
- prostaglandins to ripen the cervix. this makes it soft and thin so it can open more easily. often a gel or strip that goes into the vagina, or a pill taken by mouth.
- devices to ripen and dilate the cervix, such as a catheter to put pressure against it or a tiny rod that expands and stretches it open.
- breaking your bag of waters (with a tiny hole) to make contractions start or get stronger.
- medicines (like pitocin) that make contractions start or get stronger.

People who have labor induced have a higher chance of needing a c-section. Your provider may feel it is worth this risk if you or your baby have medical problems. These might be an infection, your bag of waters is low on fluid, you or baby has blood pressure problems or baby has stopped growing as they should.

Pain medicine

Giving birth is hard work and drugs have limits. There is no way to make birth painless. Pain medicines (drugs) can help with some of the pain, but not all of it.

It is good to learn how to manage pain and to practice ways to relax. Labor tends to go faster if you wait as long as you can before taking a drug. So, even if you want pain medicine, you will still need to cope with some pain in the earlier parts of labor. Also, drugs don't always work as quickly or as well as you want them to.

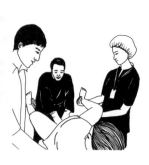

Kinds of pain medication

Learn about what kinds of pain relief there are, when they can be used, and their side effects. At a prenatal checkup, ask your provider what kinds of drugs they prefer to use and why. Tell your partner and provider what you would like to use and put it in your birth plan.

Different kinds of drugs are used depending on:

◆ how you are doing.

◆ how baby is doing.

◆ what progress you have made in labor.

These drugs usually are very safe, but may have some side effects. It is important to know the risks before you agree to use any drug. Ask your provider about the side effects before labor starts. Think about your options now, since it's hard to make decisions when you're in labor.

◆ **Pain drugs** are narcotics. You feel less pain but still feel the peak of each contraction and the urge to push. Pain drugs cannot be used in the pushing stage because they may affect baby's breathing. They might make you feel dizzy, itchy, or like throwing up.

- **Sleep aids** may help you rest in the early stage of labor. They may help you relax if you are nervous or tired. They may be given with narcotics. These drugs may affect your baby as well as you.

Epidural or spinal block to numb belly and below

An epidural or spinal block make the lower part of your body numb so it doesn't feel pain (see picture). For a spinal block, drugs are put into your lower back with a needle. For an epidural, a large needle is used to place a very narrow tube into the space around your spinal cord in your lower back. Drugs are given through this tube. You will feel little to no pain or urge to push.

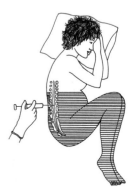

An epidural numbs the shaded area of your body.

Once you are numb, you won't be able to walk around a lot, change positions yourself, or take a bath. You will be able to push during the delivery stage, but you won't feel the contractions. Your provider or a nurse will feel your uterus. When it gets hard, they will tell you to push.

In some cases, an epidural or spinal block makes labor go quicker. In other cases, it slows labor down. It may make a c-section more likely. Also, there can be side effects for you afterwards, such as a bad headache. It is, however, good to know that the drugs used affect baby less than other kinds of drugs.

Episiotomy – A cut through your perineum

Pushing baby through the skin around your vagina is hard work. A cut or episiotomy (ep-easy-oto-me) can be done to make a bigger opening for baby to come through.

Most people do not need episiotomies, but some providers do them often. In most births, the perineum will stretch on its own, but this takes time. Some providers want to do it to speed things up. Many people don't want to be cut because they:

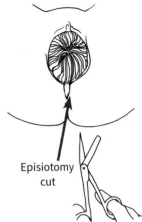

Episiotomy cut

- don't want to have to care for the cut and stitches.
- have learned that a tear often heals faster.
- worry about other health problems it could cause later.

If you do not want an episiotomy, tell your provider and put that in your birth plan. Ask your birth partner to remind your provider during birth.

If there are problems as the baby is coming out, you might need an episiotomy. Ask your provider if they think it is really needed. If it is, they will make the area numb so you do not feel the cut or the stitches afterward.

It is hard to prevent tearing during pushing. But, these things may help:

- Push in positions that open your pelvis, such as squatting or kneeling.

- Ask your provider to put a warm wet cloth on the area during pushing.

- Try to relax and slow down your pushes when your provider tells you to.

Forceps and vacuum extractors

Some babies need help getting all the way through the birth canal. This can happen if you get too tired to push harder or if baby gets stuck in the pelvis. Your provider may have tools they can use to help you avoid a surgical birth.

Forceps are large tongs that fit over baby's head. A **vacuum extractor** has a suction cup that attaches to the top of baby's head. Both are tools that let your provider pull on baby while you push during contractions.

Using these tools does have some risk, but they also help prevent bigger risks. If your provider feels it's urgent to get baby the rest of the way out quickly, one of these tools may be the safest thing. If they don't work, a c-section would need to be done.

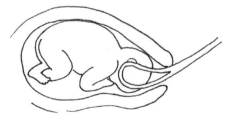

Forceps

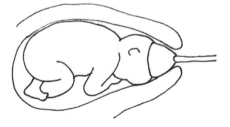

A vacuum extractor

Breech birth – Baby's head is not down

Some babies start labor lying with head forward, head up, or sideward. Sometimes it is possible for baby to flip over during labor. Your provider may try to get baby to move by pressing on the outside of your belly. You can try getting down on hands and knees or into another position that makes space for baby to turn.

If baby will not turn, your provider will talk to you about next steps. Vaginal births for breech babies can be very risky. When baby is born head first, it is easier for the narrower parts of baby to come out. When baby comes bottom or feet first, the head or shoulders can get stuck in the pelvis.

While vaginal breech births can be done safely, there are fewer and fewer providers who know how to do them. Most breech births are done by c-section because the risks are much lower for you and baby. See pages 133 and 134 for how to get baby to turn before birth.

Cesarean section – Surgical birth

A cesarean section, often called a **c-section**, is when baby is born through abdominal (belly) surgery. It may be planned ahead of time, done after a very long labor that stalls, or used to save a life in an emergency. A c-section does have serious risks, but it can be the safest way for baby to be born in some cases.

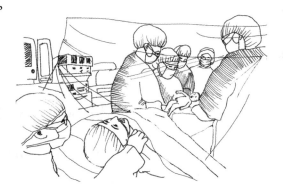

What is it like? – Getting ready

C-sections happen in an operating room with lots of doctors and nurses wearing gowns, hats, and masks. The room will have bright lights and lots of medical machines.

You will have an IV port (small needle that tubes can connect to) in your arm for medicines and fluids. You will wear an oxygen tube under your nose and a blood pressure cuff on your arm. They will put stick-on sensors on your chest to watch how your heart is doing throughout surgery. They will also put a catheter (a tiny tube) into your urethra to keep your bladder empty during surgery. Your pubic hair may be trimmed. Your legs may be put in special sleeves that massage your legs to prevent blood clots.

What is surgery like?

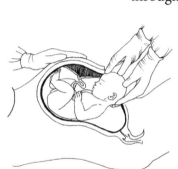

There will be an anesthesiologist (an-uhs-thee-zee-ol-uh-jist) nearby making sure your numbing medicines are working well. Your partner may be able to be with you when it's time for baby to be born.

You will be mostly numb from the top of your waist down to your feet (see epidurals, pg. 167). You may feel tugging, but you should not feel sharp pain. Once you are numb, your belly will be washed and a sheet will be hung above your chest, between you and the doctors. You may ask if you can have a sheet you can see through so you can see baby being born.

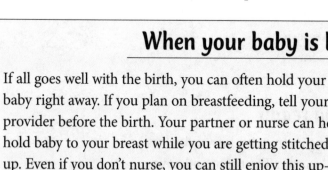

The doctor will make a cut just above your pubic hair and make a path through tissue and around muscle to get to your uterus. They may use some tools to help hold your belly open and protect your other organs. Then, they will make another cut into the uterus. The baby is pulled out by hand and fluid is suctioned from their nose and mouth. The umbilical cord is clamped and cut and baby is quickly checked before you meet them. This part often takes about 10 minutes.

When your baby is born

If all goes well with the birth, you can often hold your baby right away. If you plan on breastfeeding, tell your provider before the birth. Your partner or nurse can help hold baby to your breast while you are getting stitched up. Even if you don't nurse, you can still enjoy this up-close skin-to-skin time with baby.

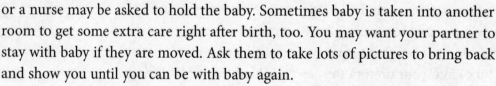

It can take a few hours for your drugs to wear off. If you're not feeling well or need extra care, your partner or a nurse may be asked to hold the baby. Sometimes baby is taken into another room to get some extra care right after birth, too. You may want your partner to stay with baby if they are moved. Ask them to take lots of pictures to bring back and show you until you can be with baby again.

Once baby is born, the placenta is taken out of your uterus. The doctor stitches the cut in your uterus closed and carefully guides your organs and muscles back into place. The cut in your belly is closed, using stitches, glue, or staples. This part can take up to an hour.

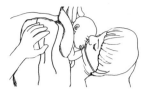

You can ask to hold baby and even breastfeed right after surgery.

What is recovery like?

Surgical births can sometimes have a hard recovery. It can take a few hours for your medicines from surgery to wear off. You will stay in the hospital for about 2–4 days. This gives you time to rest and have lots of help when you need to get up to walk. You will have some cramps and bleeding (it might feel like a heavy period). You may also have some pain and numbness near your incision (cut from surgery). Your provider will check for signs of infection, heart problems, or too much bleeding. They will also make sure you can pee after the catheter is removed. You will keep getting fluids through your IV until you can eat and drink. You will also have pain medicine to keep you comfortable.

At home, you will need to keep resting so your belly can heal. Your provider will talk to you about how active to be and how to do it safely. They will tell you how to take care of your incision and how to watch for infection. They'll give you tips on how to be gentle with your belly, like how to protect it while pushing poop out in the week or so after birth.

"They told me not to lift anything heavier than my baby for the first week. I couldn't even lift her car seat."

See chapter 16 for more on postpartum recovery.

Reasons for a c-section

There are risks with a c-section, for both you and baby. But in some cases, it is still the safest way for baby to be born.

If your provider learns of a problem in pregnancy that makes a vaginal birth unsafe, they may want to plan ahead for a c-section. This could include:

- baby is breech (bottom down) and won't turn.
- the placenta or cord is not in a good position or is blocking baby's way out.
- if you have had a c-section before (see VBAC on page 174).

A c-section may also be needed if problems come up during labor or birth. This could include:

- very high blood pressure (**preeclampsia**).
- herpes sores near vagina when labor starts.
- baby's position or size has made them stuck.
- active labor has stopped and won't get going.
- baby shows signs of stress and their heart rate is too low or too high.

Risks of a c-section

Be sure to talk about the possible risks of this surgery before you choose or agree to have one.

Some serious problems that can happen to you are:

- a bad reaction to the numbing medicines.
- injury to your bladder or bowel.
- more bleeding than normal.
- blood clots that can harm your heart or lungs.
- wound infection.
- death (very rare but more likely compared to vaginal birth).

Some serious problems that can happen to baby are:

- breathing problems at birth.
- a hard time learning to nurse.
- asthma or allergies in the future.
- death (very rare)

Benefits of a c-section

Surgical birth does have good sides to it, too. They can:

- avoid certain risks of a vaginal birth.
- help you know when and how long birth will be.
- let you plan ahead for time off of work and extra help at home.
- make it more likely for your doctor to be the one who does it.

These can be helpful to keep in mind if you need to have a c-section. They can also help you compare the risks versus the benefits (pros and cons) if you are still trying to decide.

Elective c-section – Surgery by choice

People want surgical births for many reasons. If there is no medical reason to have a c-section, a vaginal birth is often the safest choice. But there are other reasons people choose surgical birth that still may make it the best option for them. If you feel like this, talk to your provider about why. They will look at your risk factors and make sure you know the risks to you and baby. This includes more risks if you try to have more children. Knowing all of that, you can then make the choice that feels right for you.

If you do choose to plan a c-section, your provider will help you choose how to do it as safely as possible. Most babies have fewer problems if they stay in until full term. So, your surgery will likely be planned in the 39th week.

But I didn't want a c-section

It is often hard when birth doesn't go as you had hoped. If you wanted a vaginal birth but end up needing surgery, you may have some big feelings. Even if you are glad your baby is here safely, you may still be sad, or even mad, that your plans changed. It's okay to have mixed feelings.

Talk to your providers about what is important to you. Many other parts of your birth plan may still be possible, like:

- playing music or having the lights dimmed.
- seeing baby be born or pulling them up onto your chest yourself.
- having partner say baby's sex or cut the cord.
- putting baby skin to skin on your chest for bonding or nursing.
- having birth photos taken.

See page 174 for more on coping when birth doesn't go as planned.

Vaginal birth after cesarean (VBAC)

Many people want to have a vaginal birth with their next child. They may not want surgery, or to take such a long time healing. Or, they may just want to know what a vaginal birth is like.

For most people, VBAC is a safe choice. The risks of complications are very low. Some people worry that the uterus will tear where it was cut before. This is called uterine rupture, and it is very rare. But for others, the risks are higher. Talk to your doctor or midwife. They will look closely at how and why your c-section was done and any other risks for you and baby. Ask them about the risk of a VBAC compared to the risk of another c-section. You can also ask another provider what they think (this is called getting a second opinion).

If your risks are low, your provider may suggest a trial of labor after cesarean (TOLAC). This means that your provider will watch you very closely for signs of danger for you or baby. Most people who try for a VBAC are able to have one. But if there is any sign of danger, it may be safest to switch to a surgical birth.

When things don't go as planned

What if baby comes too fast to get to my provider?

Sometimes a baby might start to come out before you can get to the hospital or birth center. This is more likely if it is *not* your first baby. If you feel like you want to push or there's something in your vagina, call 911 right away.

> This guide does not replace help from paramedics or instructions from a health care provider by phone.

If your baby starts to come out before you get to the hospital:

1. Call 911 right away. Medics know how to deliver babies.
2. Do what the person on the phone tells you to do until helps gets there. (You also could call your doctor or midwife so they know what's happening.)
3. Do not try to drive to the hospital. If you are in the car, stop in a safe place. Lean your seat back or lie on the back seat. Put a clean cloth under your bottom.

4. If baby comes out before medics arrives, wipe their face and dry their head. Do not pull on the cord or cut it.

5. Keep baby dry and warm, on your bare chest. Dry baby's body, rubbing their back to help them breathe. Cover both of you with a blanket, coat, or sweater. Cover baby's head (but not face) to keep them warm.

6. Push out the placenta. Keep it for the doctor to see.

7. Put baby to your breast and try to nurse.

8. Get medical help as soon as possible.

What if baby is born early?

A baby born in the 37th or 38th week is called early term. Early term babies usually do well after birth, but may need some extra care at first. This is why most babies should not be born until at least 39 weeks.

A baby born earlier than 37 weeks is called **preterm** or **premature** (a "**preemie**"). Twins and multiple babies often come early. Some preemies just need time to grow bigger. Others needs lots of extra care so they can grow like they would have in the uterus. Many tiny babies grow up healthy and live long lives.

A preemie who needs a lot of care would be taken to a special care nursery (newborn intensive care unit or NICU*). They would be kept in a special covered bed (**incubator** or **isolette**) to keep warm. This might be at another hospital.

*NICU is pronounced "nick-you."

If this happens, try to spend as much time there as you can. Your baby needs to hear your voice and feel your touch even if they are very tiny. When possible, try to hold baby against your skin, called **kangaroo care** (chapter 11).

Get help using a breast pump so you can get your milk flowing. You will be able to bring your milk to the NICU for when baby's well enough to have it. (See chapter 11 for more about preemies.)

What if baby is very small?

Some babies born after 37 weeks are smaller than normal, under 5½ pounds (2500 grams). This is called a low-birthweight (LBW) baby.

A baby may be small because of health problems. LBW babies often need extra special care, like a preemie. With good care, most will get healthy and live long lives.

Your feelings after birth

Many people spend a lot of time thinking about what their birth will be like and how they want it to go. You may have felt strongly about letting labor start on its own, not using pain medicine, or having a vaginal birth. If any of these things don't happen the way you planned, you may feel very sad, let down, or even mad.

These feelings are normal. It is important that you and your baby are healthy, but that doesn't make the other feelings go away. Some people feel like they failed or think their body is broken. These feelings can be very hard to talk about. They can make you feel guilty. Remember, it's okay and normal to feel disappointed. It doesn't mean you don't love your baby.

Share your feelings with someone who understands. Find a support group or a counselor. It is very helpful to be with other parents who have felt how you feel. Write your feelings down. It helps to work through your feelings so you can heal. Then you can focus on being a great parent to your beautiful baby.

My baby's birth day!

My baby's name is _____

Baby was born on _____ at _____

DATE   AM / PM

Weight: _____ pounds/kg   Length: _____ inches

Head size (how big around): _____ inches

First sign of labor: _____

_____

I got to the hospital/birth center on _____ at _____

DATE   AM / PM

I was in labor for _____ hours.

Things I did that helped labor go well _____

_____

_____

My birth partner(s) helped by: _____

_____

My nurses, doctor, or midwife helped by: _____

_____

Pain medicine I was given, if any _____

How I felt right after birth _____

_____

_____

Notes from my birth partner _____

_____

_____

Notes from my doctor or midwife _____

_____

_____

_____

_____

Chapter 11

Caring for Your New Baby

Now your baby is born. You can finally see and hold them. What an exciting time!

Once your baby begins to breathe, they are living on their own. They are no longer protected by the uterus. Loud noises and bright lights are new, and the cooler air of the room could be a shock. Snuggling baby against your skin is a good way to help them feel at home. Letting baby nurse will give you both a feeling of closeness.

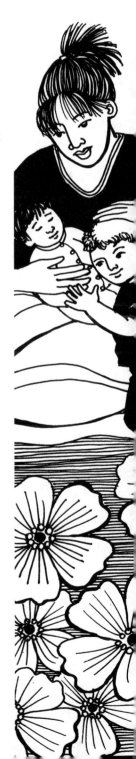

This and the following chapters will cover the basics.

Your new baby's health

Your provider will check your baby to make sure they are doing well. Most of this can be done with baby on your chest or nursing. In the first few minutes after birth, your provider will check baby's:

- heart rate.
- breathing and skin color.
- temperature.
- muscles and reflexes.
- weight and length.

Soon after, your provider will want to:

Hold baby or nurse baby during shots or blood draws. It will help baby feel less pain.

- give baby a shot of vitamin K to prevent bleeding problems.
- put medicine in baby's eyes to prevent infection.
- draw some blood from baby's heel for a "newborn screen." The blood will be tested to check for some rare but very serious problems. Often a second screen is done after a week. This is important to catch any problems that might have been missed the first time.
- take blood for a **jaundice** (**bilirubin**) screening.
- test baby for heart problems.
- check baby's hearing.

It's okay to ask questions about any of these things before they are done.

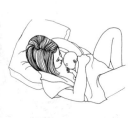

It is good for baby to be on your bare skin. You'll be covered up to keep both of you warm. The nurse or midwife may offer to clean baby up and put a diaper and hat on them. If all is well, you can hold and nurse baby as long as you want. They don't need a bath right away. The white **vernix** helps their skin stay healthy.

Welcome your baby

Many newborn babies are wide awake for a few hours after birth and then take a long nap. When baby sleeps, you should try to nap too.

After birth you may feel very emotional. Some parents feel great love for their babies right away. Others can't believe the birth has really happened. Some are too tired or sore to be able to focus on baby. Many parents look at their brand new baby and wonder how they will be able to take care of such a tiny person. All of these feelings are normal right now. All of these feelings are normal and will get better. Try to rest whenever you can and make sure you eat, too.

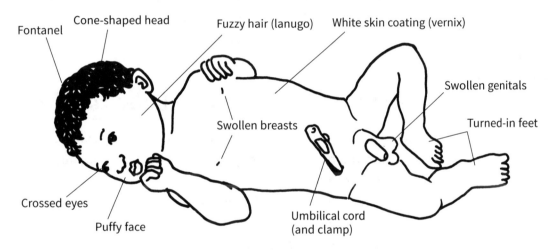

Fontanel
Cone-shaped head
Fuzzy hair (lanugo)
White skin coating (vernix)
Swollen genitals
Turned-in feet
Swollen breasts
Crossed eyes
Puffy face
Umbilical cord (and clamp)

What a newborn baby looks like

Your brand new baby

A baby who has just been born looks very different from a baby who is even a month old. A newborn will change a lot in the first few weeks.

Your baby's face may seem puffy. Their eyes may be swollen and may look cross-eyed. If you had a vaginal delivery, baby's head is likely to be cone-shaped and have a flat nose. This is from being squeezed coming through the birth canal. All of these things are normal and should go away.

Your baby's skin may have a reddish color, with little white spots (**milia**) on their nose, cheeks, and chin. The creamy white coating (**vernix**) on their skin at birth may stay in the folds of their skin. There may be fine, soft hair on their back and face (**lanugo**). Their skin may be dry and peeling. One or both feet may be turned in. Their hands and feet may look blue or purple and feel cool. All of these things are normal and should get better soon. Lots of babies are born with red, brown, or even blue or gray birth marks. Scratches or bruises from birth will heal.

Baby's head will have two soft spots called **fontanels**. These are places where the bones of the skull have not grown together yet. If you press gently, you can feel a large one on the top and a small one on the back. The fontanels will close slowly by about 18 months of age. A strong layer under the skin protects the brain.

*labia: "lips" below the vulva that close to cover up the opening of the vagina

**scrotum: pouch of skin that holds the testicles that hang below the penis.

Your baby's genitals may not look as you expect. A newborn's labia* are often swollen and spread apart. A newborn boy's scrotum** is often swollen. Their penis may look odd to you if you have not seen an intact (not circumcised) penis.

Amazing things a new baby can do

Your new baby can see things that are up close. They can see your face when you hold them. They hear and like calm, soft, high voices. They can taste and smell.

Your baby's body moves on its own in some ways. These are called reflexes. These will go away in a few weeks or months. Watch for these reflexes now:

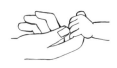

- ◆ When you touch the palm of their hand, they will hold your finger tightly.
- ◆ If you stroke their cheek, they will turn their head and open their mouth (rooting).
- ◆ When they hear a loud sound, they will startle (jerk suddenly).
- ◆ If you hold them up with their feet touching a table, they will lift up one foot (like stepping).

The first day

New baby care is very simple: keep your baby warm, fed, comforted, and clean. Your nurse, midwife, or doula can help you learn these basics before you have to do them alone. It will take a little practice to feel you know what to do. Your baby will be okay while you learn. The most important thing is to be gentle and loving with your baby.

Feeding your newborn

Your baby knows how to suck. They have been sucking their fingers in the uterus. Offer your breast right after birth. Baby may want to latch on right away. But, it is also normal if baby doesn't want to nurse very much at first.

The nurses or a breastfeeding expert (lactation consultant) can help you get started. If you have questions, or feel unsure, be sure to ask before you go home.

To get breastfeeding off to a good start:

◆ Hold your baby so their tummy is against yours.

◆ Touch their top lip with your nipple.

◆ Make sure their mouth is wide open and both lips are out. The nipple and most of the dark areola will fit inside.

◆ Let baby nurse often. Their stomach is too small to hold much milk at once.

◆ Ask the nurses not to give them water or formula. That will make baby less hungry for your milk.

If you bottle feed, give only very small amounts at first. Newborns have very small stomachs. Eating too much can cause problems.

For a whole chapter on feeding, read chapter 12.

Ways to hold and comfort baby

◆ **Cuddling:** Babies love to be held. Cuddle your baby against your chest so they can hear your heart beat, feel your warmth, and smell your body. Gently pat or rub their back.

◆ **Kangaroo care (skin to skin):** Your new baby may like being held with their skin against your bare chest. Put a light blanket over both of you. Skin-to-skin care is especially good for preemies and can help them develop well. This closeness also helps get your milk supply started.

- ◆ **Moving:** Babies love to be rocked and walked. It gives them the same feeling they had in your belly. Remember to keep one hand behind baby's head. They're not strong enough to hold up their heavy head for long.

- ◆ **Sounds:** Babies like high, sing-song sounds. They like the beat of songs. Talk to your baby in a soft voice. This kind of baby talk is natural and helps them learn. You can use real words or gentle sounds.

- ◆ **Sucking:** Babies suck for comfort, even when they're not hungry. Offer a clean finger or knuckle, or a pacifier.

Read Chapter 13 to learn more about baby.

Circumcision

If your baby has a penis, you will need to decide if you want them circumcised or not. If you want it, it is done soon after birth, so it's good to decide before baby comes.

What is circumcision surgery like?

At birth, the skin on the penis covers all the way over the tip. Circumcision is a minor surgery that cuts part of the skin off to uncover the tip of the penis. It does hurt, but they can use medicines to help.

After surgery, you must take care of the cut while it heals. This usually takes about a week. There are small chances of infection or other problems.

Why or why not to circumcise?

Some parents choose to circumcise due to religious beliefs or because they value the health benefits later on. Others choose not to circumcise because they don't want their baby to have painful surgery. Many want their child's penis to look like their dad's or look the same as other kids in school.

There are health benefits of circumcising, but they are not many. Talk to your provider and ask questions. You may also want to find out if it's covered by your insurance. Decide what feels right to you and your partner.

Baby care basics

Keep baby warm

New babies are used to the warmth of your body. Baby may need one more layer than what you're wearing to stay warm. Long sleeves and socks or adding a swaddle is often enough.

"My baby's hands are always cool, so I check their tummy to see if they're cold."

Baby could get too hot if bundled up too much. See page 193 on how to dress baby for warm or cold weather.

Swaddling

Your baby may like being wrapped snugly in a thin blanket. (See pictures below.) Swaddling helps baby feel warm and safe, just like in the belly. Wrap snugly around baby's back. You can leave their hands in or out. Leave the bottom loose so their legs can move. **Baby's arms should be out of their swaddle before they can roll over (2 to 3 months old).**

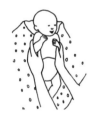 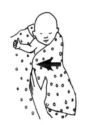 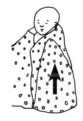 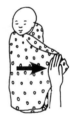 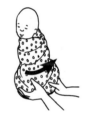

1. Place baby's head at one corner of a thin blanket.

2. Bend the knees, then wrap one corner around and tuck it in.

3. Pull the bottom corner to baby's chest. You can leave arms in or out.

4. Wrap the other corner around and tuck it in.

5. Baby's legs should be able to move freely.

Swaddling your baby with feet loose

Keep baby clean

Change your baby's diaper often to protect their tender skin. Some babies cry when they are being changed. They may feel old when they are naked.

It is good to check baby's diaper often. Wet diapers tell you baby is getting enough breast milk or formula. Once feeding is going well, they should have at least six to eight wet diapers each day.

Your newborn's first few stools (poops) are thick and black. This is called **meconium** and it is normal. The next few poops will be greenish. After that, they will be yellow. Baby probably will have three to four dirty diapers a day at first.

Be sure to wash your hands well with soap before and after each diaper change.

Keep germs away

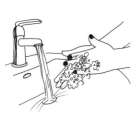

Wash your hands often when caring for your baby. Make sure that others who care for baby also wash their hands first. Even if hands look clean, they can carry germs.

Keep your new baby away from people with colds or other illnesses baby might catch. It's best not to take your baby into crowds, such as stores or parties, until they are older. This is especially important if baby is a preemie or has any breathing problems.

Keep baby safe

The most important safety concerns with new babies are injury in car crashes and during sleep. Sleep problems include Sudden Infant Death Syndrome (SIDS) and suffocation*.

*Suffocation:
Breathing blocked by pillow, quilt, cushions, or position against a wall.

Sleep safety basics:

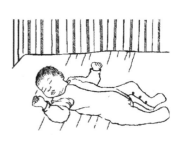

- Always put your baby to sleep on their back unless there is a medical reason not to.
- Have baby sleep in the same room with you but in their own safe bed (crib or bassinet).
- Use a firm mattress and keep pillows, quilts, and toys out of the crib.
- Dress them warmly and keep the room comfortably cool. Baby should be warm but not hot.
- Keep them away from smoky places.
- Breastfeed them.
- Give a pacifier for sleep. (Do not force or prop it in.)

Car safety basics:

- Make sure to use a car seat on every car ride.
- Install the car seat tightly in the back seat, facing the back of the car.
- Buckle the harness (straps) over each shoulder and between their legs.
- Make straps snug.

For many important details about safety, read chapter 14.

Before you take your baby home

- Know whom to call if you or your baby has a health problem.
- Get the name and phone number of a breastfeeding expert (lactation consultant).
- Make sure your baby has started to breastfeed well. Know how to get them to suck on the nipple and areola (latch on) properly. Practice squeezing (expressing) a small amount of milk out of your nipples with your fingers.
- Buckle your baby's car seat into the back seat for the ride home. Take off swaddling blankets before putting baby in the car seat.
- Make an appointment to bring your baby for their first checkup. This is usually between one and three days after going home.

Going home

If both you and your baby are doing well, you will probably be able to go home within a day or two after delivery. Being at home will give you more rest and keep you away from germs.

If you have had a c-section, you will need to stay longer to recover. If your baby is very small or had problems at birth, they will probably have to stay longer, too.

Make the first ride a safe ride

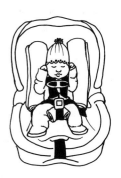

One of the most important things is to get baby buckled into their seat properly. If you have a seat with a handle, you can buckle up baby inside your room. Then carry baby in it to the car. If the seat has a base or is a convertible, install that in the car first.

Take off any blankets. Slide baby's bottom all the way back in the seat. Put the straps up over each shoulder. Pull the bottom of the straps over each hip so the pieces of the buckle are between baby's legs. Buckle both sides of the straps at the crotch and at the chest clip. Pull straps snug and make sure the chest clip points to the armpits.

If you take a taxi or other ride home, be sure the driver gives you time to get the car seat properly installed, following the instructions.

Support from your health care providers

"I wasn't sure if I should call about baby's runny nose, but the nurse told me 'There's no such thing as a dumb question!'"

You can get support by phone or email from your providers and others, day or night. No question is too small to ask.

Make sure to have the phone numbers for support people who you can call:

- ◆ Your doctor or midwife.
- ◆ Baby's doctor or nurse practitioner.
- ◆ A lactation consultant.
- ◆ Your social worker, local family center, or new mom support group.

You may have hired a doula who will visit you and help out for the first few days or weeks. Some lactation consultants and nurses also make home visits. A home visit can be very helpful. Find out if your hospital or health department offers this service.

The first weeks at home

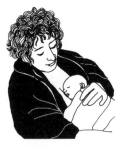

Take the time to relax with baby. Skin-to-skin time is one of the best ways to help baby feel at home in the world.

Your first days at home as a family are a very special time. It can also be a hard time. You will be tired and may feel unsure about what to do. The most important thing is to keep giving gentle, loving care to your baby and yourself.

It is also important to get as much rest as possible, so your body can heal. Try to sleep when baby does. Ask others to help you by doing laundry, cooking, grocery shopping, or cleaning. Let them do things for you and your partner so that you can pay attention to your baby.

Holding and carrying your baby

Hold baby as much as you or baby want. You can't spoil newborns. Hold your baby chest to chest or against your shoulder. Cradle baby's head by your elbow with your arm around their body. Or with their head in your hand and their body tucked near your armpit, like a football.

When your baby cries, it may mean they need something. Are they hungry, wet, tired, or lonely? You will learn which cries mean what, or if they just want to cuddle.

Wearing your baby

One way to have your baby close while you do other things is to use a cloth baby carrier. This makes it easy to take a walk, do light housework, or go shopping with your baby. This can be very soothing for a fussy baby or one who doesn't go to sleep easily.

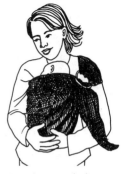

Wearing your baby.

There are many kinds of carriers. You might have to try a few before you find one that works well for you. Check how big your baby must be before using it.

Some carriers are not safe for newborns. Some require an added piece for small babies. Most carriers are not safe for small preemies, so be sure to ask baby's nurse before using one. Find one that fits your body, fits your baby, and is easy to get off and on. Find important safety tips in chapter 14.

Changing diapers

Baby's bowel movements (poops)

What goes in must come out. All parents have to clean their baby's bottom, even though it's not much fun.

Once baby's meconium has passed (see page 185), their poops will be yellow. What your baby eats can change how dark or light it is, and how it smells. Germs or tummy problems can change the texture of it.

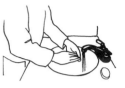

Don't forget to wash your hands after changing baby's diaper.

- ◆ Breast milk makes light yellow, very soft poops, like lumpy mustard. In the early weeks, a baby may have as many as ten small poops each day. After six weeks, baby may still poop a lot or have at least one every day or two.

- ◆ Formula makes tan or yellow poops (about as hard as peanut butter). Baby should have one or two each day.

If the poops are hard and dry, your baby may not be eating enough. Call your baby's provider.

Cleaning your baby's genitals*

*Genitals: The penis or vulva.

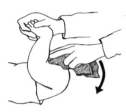

Always clean genitals from front to back.

$$ Use warm water and cotton balls or small washcloths instead of baby wipes.

Always wipe your baby's bottom from front to back. This keeps germs in the poop from getting into baby's penis or vagina. For boys, wipe the penis from base to tip. For girls, gently open the folds of skin around the vagina. Wipe them from front to back.

If your baby boy is not circumcised, the foreskin will be tight all the way to the tip. Don't try to pull it back when washing it. It will loosen itself by age 5.

A newborn girl may have some bloody or milky liquid coming from their vagina. This is normal in the first week.

Baby wipes are handy but you don't need to buy them. You can use warm water with cotton balls or small soft washcloths instead. Be sure to clean the washcloths well. It is best not to use baby oil or powder. Although they are sold for babies, they can hurt tender skin. Talcum powder can be very bad for a baby's lungs.

Care for a circumcised penis

It may take a week or two for baby's penis to heal after circumcision. Keep diapers loose. Do not lay your baby on their tummy until their penis has healed. Ask your baby's provider before you put any ointment or a bandage on it.

To keep the area clean, wash it very gently when changing diapers. Drip warm soapy water over it. Rinse it with warm clean water and then pat it dry.

Call the doctor or nurse if you see bleeding or signs of infection. Infection causes pus, redness, and swelling. Also call if your baby has a hard time peeing.

Diaper rash

*Diaper rash: A painful, red, bumpy rash around the genitals and bottom.

Baby's skin is very thin. It can get irritated when it has pee or poop on it for too long. This is called diaper rash*, and it is very common. Here are some tips to avoid it:

- Change your baby's diaper every two or three hours and as soon as possible after each bowel movement.
- Dry the area well with a cloth or air dry.

- Let your baby lie without a diaper on for a while every day.

- Smear oil (like olive or coconut) or petroleum jelly (like Vaseline) all over baby's bottom before putting on a new diaper.

When your baby has a rash, change their diaper more often. Follow all of the "how to avoid diaper rash" steps above. These will help it hurt less and help it heal.

If baby gets rashes often, or if they get very raw or last more than a few days, talk to baby's provider. They can make sure it's not infected and help figure out the cause.

"I give baby naked bum time during tummy time and it helps so much. I just put socks and a shirt on them or turn the heat up."

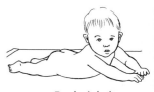

Fresh air helps prevent and calm diaper rash.

Cord care in the first few weeks

Keep the cord stump clean and dry. Fold the front of each clean diaper down below the stump. Clean the area around the stump with warm water once a day and if it gets stool on it. Do not put baby's belly under water until a few days after the stump falls off. The stump will get dry and black. It may start to smell bad, too. Never try to pull it off. It will fall off in about a month and will leave a nice belly button.

If the skin around the stump gets red, hot, or oozes pus, call your baby's provider. They can make sure it's not infected and tell you how to help it.

Bathing your new baby

Young babies don't need full baths often. Baby's face, hands, neck, and bottom should be wiped clean three times a week. This is called a **sponge bath**. You may also check baby's folds, like in their armpits and thighs. Follow care tips for their belly button and circumcision, as needed. As baby gets older, you may give baby baths in the water.

For a happy and safe bath time:

- Have all supplies right next to bath: Wash cloth, mild soap, towels, small cup, and a diaper.

- Make sure room is warm. Have towels ready.

- Use water that is warm to your wrist or elbow, but not too hot.

- Start with baby's face and head, then down to neck, end with baby's bottom.

♦ **Never let go of baby, even for a second!** Even if you have a bath seat.

Swaddle baby for bath time

Wrapping baby in a thin blanket or towel can keep them warm and calm at bath time. It also makes it easy to hold onto them. No matter how you bathe baby, **always start with their face and head**. As you move down their body, you open the swaddle to uncover the part you want to wash. When it's clean, you cover it back up.

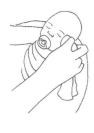 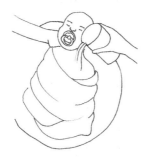 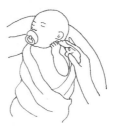 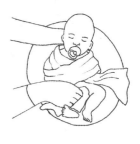

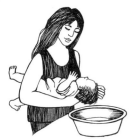

Washing baby's hair.

Sponge bath – Baby not in the water

A **sponge bath** is when you use a wet cloth to wipe baby clean without putting them in the water. You may want to do it on a wide counter or a table. Have a soft wash cloth (not a sponge) and two bowls of warm water. One bowl is for washing, so you can put a bit of mild soap in it. The other bowl is to rinse your cloth between body parts.

Tub bath – Baby in the water

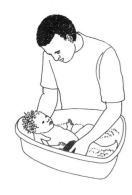

After baby's cord stump falls off, you can put baby in the water for baths. You can use a clean sink, large bowl, or a small baby tub. If baby does not like it, try swaddling baby (see above) or laying a large washcloth on their chest. Use a cup to pour water over their chest often to keep them warm.

♦ Have all bath supplies right next to bath.
♦ Hold baby with one arm wrapped under their head and neck. Hold their arm or armpit with that hand.
♦ Wash and rinse with your other hand.
♦ Never let go of baby in the bath—even for a second! A baby can drown quickly and silently if their face goes in the water.

Baby's skin

A new baby's skin may get very dry. This is normal and usually okay left alone. If you are worried that baby's skin is too dry, you can rub on a mild, unscented skin cream.

Rashes are common in babies, and are usually normal. You can try using soaps that are not scented for baby's skin and laundry.

Some babies have tiny pimples on their face and body. This is also normal and will go away. Don't try to scrub or pop them, and don't use any special soaps or creams.

You may see small brown or yellow flakes under baby's hair. This is called **cradle cap** and is very common. Wash baby's hair normally. You may also use a soft brush after bath, but don't scrub or pick the scales off. Some oils can make it worse and picking can harm baby. If it bothers you or baby, talk to baby's provider about how to help it clear.

If your baby has any rash, bumps, or dry spots that seem to be itchy or painful, talk to their provider. Call if you see anything that turns bright red, bleeds, or oozes yellow pus.

"My baby loved to be massaged with oil. It was a little game we played after a bath. I'd tell them how cute their tummy, fingers, and toes were."

Cleaning gums and teeth

Most babies do not get their first teeth until at least four months. Before teeth start coming in, it is good to wipe your baby's gums with a small soft cloth every day. This helps baby get used to the feeling of having their mouth cleaned.

When baby's first teeth start coming in, wipe them daily or use a soft baby tooth brush. If you use any toothpaste, use only a tiny smear (like a grain of rice) on the brush. Ask your baby's doctor or nurse if you should use toothpaste with fluoride once your baby has their first tooth.

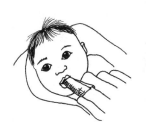

It is important to keep baby teeth healthy. Your baby needs those teeth for many things besides chewing food. Teeth help baby talk. They also hold space in the gums for the adult set of teeth.

Dressing for inside and outside

Most babies only need to wear one layer more than you do. You could put a onesie under their outfit or put them in long sleeves and socks. When outside, add a hat for warmth or sun protection. But, avoid hats in bed or in the car, as they can quickly make baby too hot.

If your baby is a preemie or under five pounds, talk to their provider about safe ways to help them stay warm.

Getting too hot is dangerous for baby. Babies can overheat from warm weather or from us bundling them up too much in the cold.

Out in warm weather, keep baby in the shade and make sure there is fresh air flow on them. Offer nursing or a bottle often and take breaks from the heat when you can.

"It snows a lot here, so I have to use a warm blanket outside. I check baby often and keep one corner flipped up to let fresh air in."

In cold weather, dress baby in thin but warm layers. Fleece pajamas, socks, booties, and hats are good ways to keep baby warm while on the go. In a car seat or stroller, a thin blanket can be folded to cover from their shoulders to their feet. The edges can be tucked snugly behind baby's arms and under their legs and feet so baby can't pull it up to their face.

Protect your baby from the sun

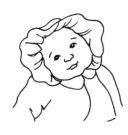

If baby's provider says that sunshine may help jaundice, ask how to do it safely.

Try to keep your baby out of direct sun for the first six months. It's very easy for baby to get sunburned, whether their skin is light or dark. Keep your baby in the shade when you can, especially between 10 a.m and 4 p.m. The sun can burn even on cloudy days. Sun is especially bright at the beach or in the snow.

When out in the sun, dress baby in thin, light-colored clothes that cover them well. Choose a sun hat with a wide brim that goes all the way around. For small areas of skin, like the face and backs of hands, use a baby sunscreen rated at least SPF 15. Reapply often.

If your baby needs special health care

Some newborn babies are born with a birth defect or a problem like low birth weight or being premature. Some problems are more serious than others.

You may never know why the problem happened. Try not to blame yourself. Instead, focus on helping baby get well.

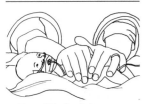

Even if baby is in an isolette, you can help by touching and talking softly to them.

If your new baby needs to stay in the hospital, they will likely be in the newborn intensive care unit (NICU). That is where baby can get the special care they need. It will have dim lights, be warm, and be as quiet as possible. These things help a baby keep growing and developing well.

While your baby is in the NICU, spend a lot of time with them if you can. Baby needs to hear your voice and feel your touch. This is as important as all the tubes, machines, and medicines. Try to help with baby's care as much as you can.

This is a good way for you and your partner to learn how to care for them when they come home.

Learn about baby's condition

- ◆ Try to be at the NICU when the doctor checks your baby. This is the best time to ask about what's happening. You also can learn a lot from the NICU nurses.

  - ▶ Find out as much as possible about the condition your baby has. Ask the hospital social worker for help getting information. See chapter 17 for resources.

  - ▶ If you are not sure a specific treatment is best for your baby, ask for a second opinion. It is always OK to ask for another doctor's advice.

Find out when "rounds" are on your unit. This is when your baby's doctors will come by each day.

Comforting your baby

Kangaroo care, holding baby skin to skin against your chest, can be very healing for your baby. It helps baby feel connected to you, breathe well, and stay calm. It also helps you bond with baby. Your partner and other family members can also do skin-to-skin care if baby's doctors allow.

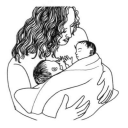

Kangaroo care
for tiny twins

Many babies can be breastfed in the NICU. But you may have to wait a few days or weeks before baby is able to nurse. Start pumping right away so your breasts will make milk. In many cases, that milk can be given to baby in a bottle until baby can nurse. Skin-to-skin time may help your milk come in during this time. Ask for a breastfeeding consultant to help you.

"When my baby was tiny, both their father and I loved holding them against our bare chests. Baby really seemed happy there."

Dealing with your feelings

If your child has a health problem at birth, it often is a big surprise. Parents whose baby is not born exactly the way they expected often feel very scared, sad, guilty, or angry. These feelings are normal. Here are some ways you can cope:

- ◆ Spend as much time as possible with your baby.

- ◆ Talk with the social worker about your feelings. The social worker can tell you about parent support groups. Partners may also want support to get through this difficult time.

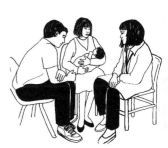

Modern medical care helps many babies with special needs to lead healthy, happy lives. Your baby will need your love and attention, just like any other baby. Caring for them can be very hard and also very rewarding.

See chapter 15 for details on caring for a sick baby.

Tips for partners

- **Touch your baby.** Hold them, talk to them, let them sleep on your bare chest. This is good for baby and will help you feel connected.

- **Support your partner.** They may be very emotional, with good feelings or with worries. Be kind and loving.

- **Help care for baby.** Change diapers, learn to swaddle or get baby dressed. Be the master of burping or giving baths. Rock or walk with your baby while your partner rests.

- **Talk to baby's provider.** You can help by asking questions. You can make notes of what the doctor, nurse, or midwife says. Help by keeping track of paperwork and phone numbers.

- **Let people help.** These first weeks are hard. Tell people what they can do. Let them bring you meals, walk the dog, or mow the lawn. Let them help you, so you can help your partner and baby.

- **Take pictures now.** The first months go by so quickly. Your baby will change before your eyes. Make sure you have photos to remember this special time.

Chapter 12

Feeding Your New Baby

Your most important job

Feeding time is special. It's not just about filling baby's tummy. It's also about baby feeling connected to someone. Baby will be happiest if they are fed as soon as they show signs of hunger. When their needs are met quickly, baby learns to trust people.

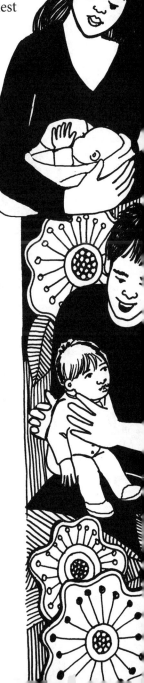

Look in this chapter for:

Baby will grow best if they are fed when they are hungry. They may eat more on some day than others. Feed baby when they start to act hungry. If you're not sure how much baby should be eating, ask their provider.

Basics of feeding from breast or bottle

Signs of hunger

Feed baby when they show signs of hunger. Try not to wait until they cry. Early signs baby is hungry may be that they:

- smack their lips or stick out their tongue.
- suck on their hand.
- make soft cooing or swallowing sounds.
- turn their head toward you when you touch their cheek.

It's important for a new baby to feed every two or three hours. Some newborns are very sleepy and need to be woken up to feed. You can wake baby gently by talking, changing their diaper, taking off some of their clothes, rubbing their back, or sitting them up.

Comfort sucking

Babies suck both for eating and for comfort. When babies comfort suck on the breast, it can help your body make more milk. But it can also make your nipples sore and make you feel stuck. Baby can also suck on their fist, your clean fingertip or knuckle, or a pacifier.

Using a pacifier

If your baby is still learning to nurse well, talk to their provider about using a pacifier. For some babies, especially preemies, a pacifier can help them learn to eat well. For others, it can make it harder. Certain shapes may be better for your baby. Or only using it at certain times like for sleep or on car rides in those first weeks.

The right pacifier can help keep baby calm and happy. It can also help keep them safe while they sleep. Just don't ever force or prop it into baby's mouth or tie it around their neck.

Get comfortable feeding

Feeding can take some time, so make sure you both are comfortable before you begin. Place a firm pillow in your lap to support your arm and your baby. Have a glass of water and a snack next to you. If you want to listen to music, make it very calm and quiet.

"Baby eats better when the room is quiet. So I turn off the TV and relax during feedings."

Pay attention to your baby at feeding time. Look in baby's eyes and smile. Talk softly or sing a song. Take this time to help baby feel safe and loved.

How do I know when baby is full?

Babies usually know when they are full. Your baby's tummy is very small and can't hold much. The first day it's as small as a cherry! By day 10, it's no bigger than an egg. That's why they need to eat so often.

Stop when your baby acts full. Giving your baby too much food will upset their tummy and be hard for both of you.

Baby is likely full if they:

- stop sucking and don't need to burp.
- turn their head away from the breast or the bottle.
- start to fall asleep.

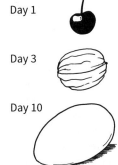

Day 1

Day 3

Day 10

A new baby's stomach is very small but grows fast.

If your baby gets sleepy after only a few minutes of feeding, try to keep them awake to finish eating. Sit baby up, burp them, or change their diaper. Then offer the nipple again. If baby still doesn't want it, wait a while.

If you are bottle-feeding, don't try to get your baby to finish a bottle. Let baby show you when they are done.

See page 209 for more on bottle feeding.

How do I know if baby's eating enough?

Feed your baby as much as they want, whenever they are hungry. You will know baby is getting enough milk if they:

- have at least six wet diapers and at least three poopy diapers every 24 hours. Their poop should be soft.
- gain weight after the first week.
- seem tired or calm after eating and burping.

"My mom told me baby would sleep better if I put cereal in baby's bottle at night. But our doctor said that's really not good for them."

A baby under 4 to 6 months of age should get enough nutrition from breast milk or formula. They should not need any other food. In fact, even water can be dangerous for babies under 6 months.

Baby can be with you at meal time. When they can sit up on their own and seem to want your food, they may be ready to try some foods. Talk to baby's provider about when to start foods.

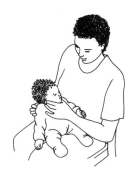

Burp baby often. Sit them in your lap and cradle their jaw in your hand and pat their back. Or try it with them lying on their tummy on your lap or up on your shoulder.

Burping is part of feeding

Babies often swallow air while eating. You may need to burp baby in the middle of a feeding and at the end.

There are lots of ways to burp a baby. You can hold your baby up by your shoulder or on your chest. You can sit them up or lay them on their tummy in your lap. Pat or rub their back gently for a few minutes. Use a cloth or small towel to catch any spit up that comes with the burp.

Warning: If your baby vomits forcefully, such that milk shoots out a few feet, baby might have a serious problem. Call the doctor or nurse right away.

Breastfeeding your baby

Breast milk is specially made for babies' needs. The milk your body makes during the first few days is especially nutritious. Your milk changes as your baby's needs change. (For more about why breastfeeding is important, see chapter 6.)

A baby does not need other foods until at least 4 to 6 months. Wait until they show interest in foods you are eating. Make sure baby can sit up and swallow well before offering other foods. The Academy of Pediatrics advises feeding only breast milk for about six months.

Most babies are ready to nurse right after birth. Many new parents love nursing their babies during the first hour or two. If you had pain medicine in labor, baby might be too sleepy to latch on at first. If this happens, don't worry. Baby will wake up and be ready to try soon. You might ask to have baby skin to skin on your chest so they can smell you.

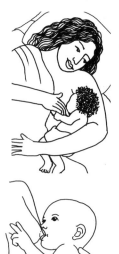

"I love that my baby looks right at me while nursing. I talk or sing to them and it helps me relax."

Help learning to breastfeed

Breastfeeding is something that you and your baby learn to do together. The most important things are that you are comfortable and have baby in a good position. This helps baby get the nipple and areola into their mouth before they start to suck. This will work better for baby and feel better for you.

Are you taking any medications or supplements? Check with your provider to make sure that if they pass to baby through your milk, it will be okay for baby.

If you are worried or in pain, ask for help. Most parents who have early nursing problems can get through them with the right help.

Who can help?

In the first few days, the nurses or your midwife will be there to help you. Many doulas have training to help you get nursing started in those first hours, too. Also ask your provider about lactation support in your area. Write down who to call if you have a problem or question later on.

There are breastfeeding educators and peer counselors who can help with common nursing struggles. Lactation consultants with "IBCLC" next to their name are certified and have the most training. They can help with more complex problems and help you know when you or baby need to see a doctor for more help.

You also can call a local breastfeeding group, such as La Leche League (see chapter 17). Leaders have lots of experience with nursing babies. Or you could find a nearby nursing support group. If you qualify for WIC, you can get breastfeeding support by phone or in person.

Making milk and nursing your baby doesn't happen easily for everyone. If you are worried or unsure, ask for help. If you don't know who to ask, call or message your insurance plan for a list of resources. All state and private plans must cover some kind of lactation support.

Making milk

Your breasts will be larger when they are making milk regularly. Your nipple and areola may also be larger and darker. Even if your breasts aren't big, they can still make plenty of milk.

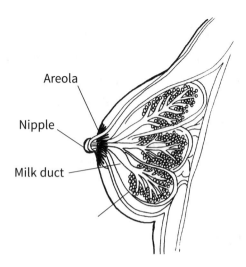

Areola

Nipple

Milk duct

Inside your breasts are the glands that make milk. They will feel like lumps all around your breast area. You may even feel them by your armpits. Tubes (ducts) carry the milk from the glands to your nipples.

After your baby starts sucking, you may feel your breasts "let down." That is when the milk starts to flow from the glands. After a few minutes, the milk gets richer. It is important to let your baby suck on each breast as long as they're still drinking and swallowing. This means they'll get the best milk. (This also is important when pumping your breasts.)

When your milk "comes in"

*Colostrum:
The first milk from
the breasts.

During pregnancy, your breasts will start to make colostrum*. It is thick and clear or yellowish. This milk is full of antibodies to protect baby from illness.

Two or three days after birth, your breasts will begin to fill with breast milk. It is white or bluish-white. It also has lots of antibodies. You may feel your breasts get full. This is normal and can last for a few days.

If they feel too full (engorged), let baby nurse more often. This will keep your breasts from getting too full. Put warm cloths on your breasts or massage them before nursing. This helps the milk flow.

If the areola gets too hard to fit into baby's mouth, you can squeeze (express) a little milk out. This will make it easier for baby to fit the nipple in their mouth.

See page 206 for more on engorged breasts.

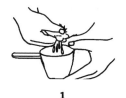

Expressing breast milk by hand.

1

Expressing milk

To express milk, press on your breast gently but firmly with your fingers. (See pictures, right.)

1. Massage from all sides toward the areola.
2. Then hold your thumb above and fingers below the areola.
3. Squeeze and release it a few times. A little milk will come out.

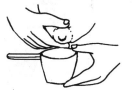

2

Once the areola is soft, baby will be able to latch on. Nursing every few hours helps keep your breasts from getting engorged.

Your breasts will feel best when your baby sucks well and empties them often. After you have been breastfeeding for a few days, they will get softer and feel more comfortable between feedings. They are getting used to making milk.

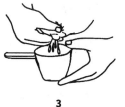

3

How often should baby eat?

- After the first day, a baby under 2 months old needs to nurse every one to three hours (eight to twelve times in 24 hours). Some may eat more often during one part of the day than another.

- If your new baby sleeps for more than four hours, it is important to gently wake them up to eat.

To know your baby is getting enough milk, make sure they are nursing often and well and seems to be happy after nursing. They should have at least six wet diapers each day. Check it often if you are concerned.

Is a disposable diaper wet? It can be hard to know. You can tell by holding it up to the light and comparing it to a dry one. Or put a piece of tissue in the diaper. The tissue will feel wet.

Ways to hold your baby while you nurse

Get comfortable. You might need to stay this way for a long time. It's good to use different positions for different feedings.

In all these positions, use pillows to make yourself and your baby comfortable. Remember to put baby's tummy flat against your body.

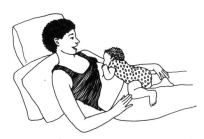

Laid-back hold: Rest against pillows. Put baby on their tummy with their head on top of your breast and their body on your tummy.

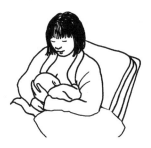

Football hold: Sit in a chair and hold your baby next to your side, with legs under your arm. Baby doesn't lie on your tummy. This is a good way to nurse if you have had a c-section.

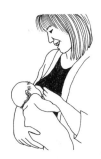

Cradle hold: Sit in an armchair. Hold your baby across your chest. Their head should be in the bend of your arm. Put a firm pillow under your baby's body and your arm.

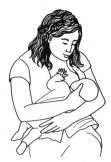

Cross-cradle hold: Sit in an armchair. Hold your baby across your chest. One hand should be at baby's head with your elbow by their bottom. Put a firm pillow under your baby's body and your arm.

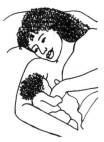

Side-lying hold: Lie in bed on your side. Lay baby on their side next to you, in the bend of your elbow or on the bed.

Basics of happy breastfeeding

Breastfeeding is natural. Once it gets going well, it can be a very happy time. Try these basic tips:

◆ Hold your baby so their tummy faces your body. Think "tummy to tummy." Baby's head should face your nipple, so they don't have to turn their head to reach it.

◆ Support your breast outside the areola with your thumb on top.

◆ Get your baby to open up wide by touching your nipple to their top lip. Open your mouth—they may do it, too.

◆ When baby's mouth is open, pull them toward you. Guide the nipple and areola deeply into their mouth.

◆ Make sure at least part of the areola gets into baby's mouth. Sucking only on the nipple will not work. Make sure their lips are curved out and the tip of their nose touches your breast. They can still breathe, just don't push the back of their head.

◆ Listen for swallowing. They will not swallow with every suck. You may hear a gulp or see the skin in front of their ears move a little.

◆ Let baby decide how long to nurse on the first breast. When their sucking slows, burp them and switch breasts. Let them nurse from both breasts at each feeding.

◆ Start the next feeding with the breast they sucked last.

◆ You might need to get the nipple out while baby is sucking. Put your finger gently into the corner of their mouth. This breaks the suction without hurting your nipple.

If your nipples start to get sore, make sure:

◆ baby is lying facing your chest.

◆ their head is not turned to the side.

◆ they have as much nipple and areola in their mouth as will fit.

◆ to get help! See chapter 17 for resources.

Nursing should not hurt. If it does, be sure to try these tips. If you still have pain, ask for help.

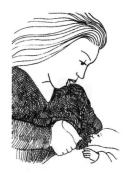

Hold your breast and pull baby to it when their mouth is wide open.

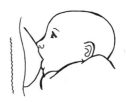

Baby's lips should be turned out.

"At first I couldn't remember which breast to begin with. Then I started clipping a little safety pin on my bra strap on the side my baby sucked last. That made life easier."

Caring for your breasts

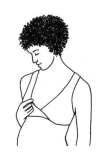

A nursing bra has flaps that open for nursing.

Nursing bras and nursing tank tops can be useful and comforting. If your breasts are heavy, find a bra that is strong enough to support them. If your breasts are small, a nursing tank top may be enough support.

Wash your breasts normally when you bathe. You don't need to wash before or after feeding. Too much soap or washing too often can make your nipples sore.

If your nipples feel sore:

- check to make sure your baby is latching on well. baby should lie with their tummy flat against your body.

- vary baby's position for different feedings. that means they will not always suck on your nipples in the same way.

- put a tiny bit of breast milk or nipple cream on your nipples after nursing. this helps healing.

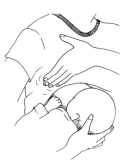

A stretchy bra may be comfortable at home or for sleep.

Engorged breasts

If your breasts get very hard (engorged), it can be painful. This can happen if you miss a feeding or stop nursing suddenly. If it lasts for more than a day or you have a fever, talk to your doctor, midwife, or a lactation consultant. Here are some ways to feel better:

- Nurse as long as your baby will suck. Let them suck all your milk out.

- Squeeze a bit of milk out before your baby latches on.

- Use a cool pack for 15 minutes after you nurse. You can put a wet washcloth in the refrigerator to cool.

- A warm wet towel might feel good.

Massaging your breasts helps the milk flow.

One way to help the milk flow through the milk glands in your breasts into the nipple is to massage your breasts gently with your fingertips as your baby sucks. This may help prevent ducts from getting blocked.

A blocked duct will feel like a sore lump in your breast. Gently massage the area and put a warm washcloth on it before nursing. Those can help the milk flow through it. Let your baby nurse on that breast first. Gently massage the lump while your baby sucks.

Call your provider or a lactation consultant right away if:

◆ a nipple cracks or starts bleeding.

◆ a duct stays blocked for two to three days.

◆ your breast has an area that is warm and painful, and you have a fever, headache, or flu-like symptoms. These are signs of mastitis*.

*Mastitis: Inflammation of the breast tissue.

Common questions

Is my baby getting enough breast milk?

Many nursing parents can make enough milk for their baby's needs. When baby is hungry, they will suck more. This tells your body to make more milk.

Every few weeks your baby will probably have a growth spurt*. When this happens, they will want to nurse more often for a couple of days. This extra nursing should boost your milk supply.

*Growth spurt: A time when baby grows faster than usual. He will suck more to get more nutrition.

Is my breast milk good enough?

Breast milk is the most nutritious milk for your baby. It has almost everything they need right now. You can make sure both you and baby get all you need by drinking lots of water and eating plenty of:

◆ calcium from dairy, leafy greens, and beans.

◆ vitamin D from sunlight and supplements.

◆ protein from meat, fish, eggs, beans, nuts, dairy.

◆ iron from meat, fish, leafy greens, fortified cereals.

◆ folic acid from leafy greens, beans, oranges, meat, and supplements.

Vitamins or supplements for baby

One thing breast milk does not have is **Vitamin D**. Vitamin D is very important as baby is growing. Our bodies make Vitamin D from the sun's rays on our skin. Baby's skin can't be in the sun for long, so this can't happen. So, all breastfed babies should take Vitamin D drops. Ask baby's provider about how much and when to start.

It is also important to have enough **iron**. Breastfed babies often need added iron around 4 to 6 months old. Talk to baby's provider about starting foods high in iron or using iron drops.

What if I didn't start nursing right after birth?

Sometimes baby can't breastfeed for a few days or weeks because of a medical problem. Usually, a baby gets breast milk from a spoon, syringe, tube, or a bottle for a few days or even a few weeks. Even if your baby must be given formula for a while, it is often possible for them to learn to nurse later.

If you can't start nursing right after birth, talk to the nurse, lactation consultant, doctor, or midwife as soon as possible. They can help you get set up to pump your breasts until your baby can nurse. Your milk is best—even during the first few days of life. So start pumping right away. If you don't pump, your breasts will stop making milk. Later, it could be very hard to get milk started.

What if nursing hurts or isn't going well?

If you are having a problem with nursing, ask for help now. Please don't just stop breastfeeding or wait until it gets worse. Call your doctor, midwife, nurse, lactation consultant, WIC clinic, or a La Leche League leader for advice. They can give you tips and support to help with most problems.

Some problems that you should call about:

- Cracked or sore nipples
- A hard, red area of your breast that feels warm
- A very sleepy baby who does not wake for feedings
- Less than six wet diapers in 24 hours

Can I breastfeed my twins?

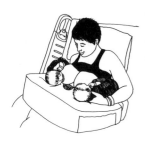

You can nurse twins, or even triplets! You may want to feed them one at a time at first. As you and the babies get used to nursing, you can feed them at the same time. This will save you a lot of time. Your breasts may make enough milk for both babies if you nurse often. It's also okay for them to have your milk at some feedings and formula at the rest.

Twins (and other multiples) are more likely to be born early or very small. They may spend time in the NICU. See page 194 to learn more.

Can I still nurse when I go back to work or school?

Breastfeeding for as long as possible is best for your baby. It also helps your body recover from pregnancy. But remember, any amount of breastfeeding is much better than not doing it at all.

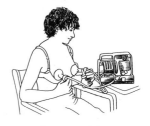

Pumping at work keeps you comfortable and gives you milk for baby.

Many parents who go back to work outside their home are able to keep breastfeeding. They look forward to the special nursing time when they get home.

To keep up your milk supply, you would use a breast pump at work. Pumping may seem strange at first, but it can give you a lot of milk quickly. The goal is to pump as many times as your baby would nurse if they were with you. Store the milk in a refrigerator or cooler. Take it home for use the next few days or freeze it for later. You can nurse your baby before you leave and when you are back.

There are pumps that you squeeze with your hand and electric pumps (see picture). Your insurance should cover an electric breast pump. WIC can also give you a pump.

"I reminded my boss that breastfed babies get sick less, which means I wouldn't need to call in sick as much."

The law says that nursing parents must have long enough breaks to pump and a private space to pump in. (A space that is not the bathroom.) Talk to your boss before you come back to work. This gives them time to find how to make it work.

Bottle feeding your baby

Whether you are using a bottle for breast milk or formula, make feeding time special. Hold your baby against your body with their head higher than their tummy. Look at baby and talk softly. Feeding time can be special, no matter how or what you're feeding your baby. Try to relax and talk or sing to your baby.

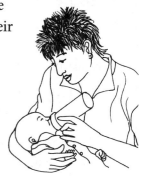

For safety, baby should always be held for feeding. Never prop a bottle in their mouth or leave them alone with it. Choking is silent and can be deadly. Make sure everyone who takes care of baby knows how to hold and feed them safely.

Become a bottle expert

Whether you are feeding breast milk or formula, be sure to:

1. use a fresh bottle for each feeding. Do not keep unused breast milk or formula to finish later. Germs can grow in the bottle, even if you keep it cold.

   Never add water to breast milk. Don't thin formula by adding more water than the directions say.

2. warm the bottle in a bowl of hot water.

   Never heat a bottle in a microwave. The milk (or formula) could get hot and burn your baby's mouth—even if the bottle does not feel hot.

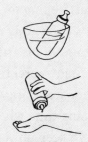

Warming a bottle and testing the temperature of milk

3. swirl or gently shake the bottle so it's all the same temperature.

4. test a little on the inside of your wrist. it should feel as warm as your skin.

5. hold baby close and a bit upright. keep baby's head higher than their bottom.

6. tap baby's top lip with the nipple. when baby opens their mouth, put the nipple in. hold the bottle so the milk fills the tip of the nipple.

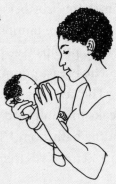

7. pause after each ounce or two. burp baby. stop when baby shows you they're full (see page 199).

8. wash the bottles and nipples in hot, soapy water after every use. Boil nipples before using for the first time.

Choosing a nipple

Newborn nipple with slow flow

- Nipples come in different shapes. your baby may like one kind better than others.

- Make sure the nipple does not flow too fast. use a newborn nipple with a small hole at first. The milk should come out slowly (see pictures). You may even try a preemie nipple.

NO!

Nipple with fast flow

Breast milk in a bottle

Many nursing parents want their baby to learn to take a bottle. This allows you to be away from home for more than an hour or two and to go back to work or school.

If baby isn't getting enough milk from nursing, you'll need to start bottle feeding early on. Even if they are nursing and peeing plenty, it's good to try bottle feeding a few weeks in. Start with just a small bit of milk in the bottle, maybe half an ounce. Offer it once or twice a day. Give baby time to get used to it. Don't wait until you're going to leave for the day to try it for the first time. Start with a preemie or newborn nipple that has a slow flow. That will be most like your breast. Hold the bottle so that the milk barely fills the tip of the nipple. This lets baby control how fast the milk comes out.

Your baby may take a bottle easier from your partner, a friend, or a grandparent. (Baby expects you to offer your breast.) If baby doesn't want the bottle, try slipping it into their mouth just as they are waking up. After a while, baby will likely learn that a bottle is just another way to get their favorite food, your milk.

Whenever your baby gets your milk from a bottle, it's best to pump your breasts. This will help your milk supply keep up. If your breasts skip a feeding, they will make less milk.

"I couldn't get my baby to take a bottle, so my friend tried. I let her hold my sleeping baby and a bottle of my milk. When baby started to wake, she slid the bottle in and they drank it! Since then, bottles have been no problem."

Using donor breast milk

Feeding your baby another person's milk can be risky. If you are worried that you aren't making enough milk, talk with your provider or a lactation consultant. Ask if any nearby hospitals have a milk bank or if there are other donor milk programs in your area. Most milk banks screen their milk (for diseases) and their donors (for risky behaviors or health problems). They also process their donor milk so you can feel sure that it's safe.

Before using any shared milk, make sure you know:

+ The health of the person it came from.
+ How clean the breast milk is.
+ How fresh it is.

Using baby formula

Some people use breastmilk and formula. Some people choose not to use any breastmilk. Some can't make or use it because of health reasons. Do not worry. Babies who are fed formula can still grow well and be very healthy.

If you are making milk but are not going to nurse or pump, you may need to stop your breasts from making milk. See page 213

Choosing a formula

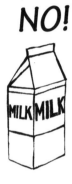

NO!

- Always use formula, not plain milk. Formula is made to be as much like breast milk as it can be. Plain cow or goat milk, soy, rice, or condensed milk **do not** have all the right nutrients for your baby. They can even cause serious problems for baby.

- Most babies do well on a formula based on cow's milk. If you think your baby has a problem with that, talk with their doctor before trying another kind.

- Choose a formula with iron unless your baby's provider tells you not to.

- Powdered formula is the least expensive but liquid, ready-to-use formula is easier. If you don't have clean water, ready-to-drink formula is best.

- If your baby is a preemie or has health issues, powdered formula may not be safe. Talk to baby's provider about what may be best.

How to use formula

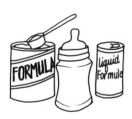

Be sure not to add too little or too much water to formula. This can be dangerous for baby.

- To mix powdered formula, follow the directions on the package. Be careful to measure correctly.

- Be sure the water is clean. If you aren't sure, use bottled water.

- While your baby is a newborn, put only a few ounces of formula in the bottle at one time. Always throw out any leftover formula after an hour.

- Do not push your baby to drink more than they want. Most babies under 2 months old only drink two to four ounces of formula every three to four hours.

◆ If you mix formula ahead of time, keep it in the refrigerator, not at room temperature. This keeps germs from growing.

How to stop making milk

If your breasts are making milk but you aren't using it, it can be painful. If you don't nurse or pump, your body will stop making milk after a week or more. If you want to stop making milk more quickly:

◆ wear a supportive bra, but don't bind (wrap) your breasts tightly.

◆ put cold (ice) packs on your breasts when they hurt.

◆ take ibuprofen or other pain relievers as needed, according to the package or your provider.

◆ if your breasts get very full and hard (engorged), you may want to express or pump just enough to make them soft. use a cold pack afterward.

◆ some people use cabbage leaves, herbs, or medicine to stop their milk. Ask a lactation consultant, nurse, doctor, or midwife before trying these things.

Tips for partners

◆ Encourage your partner to breast feed as long as they can. It's healthy for baby and you don't have to pay extra money for formula.

◆ Take the lead when it's time for baby to learn to drink from a bottle. If baby is still nursing, they are more likely to take a bottle from you than your partner.

◆ Once baby knows how to drink from a bottle, offer to feed baby. Give your partner a break by taking over a night feeding or sending them out for a few hours.

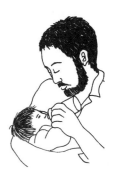

◆ Burp the baby! If your partner nurses, hold and burp baby while your partner switches breasts. When baby is done nursing, take them for a good burping.

Chapter 13

Getting to Know Your Baby

A newborn baby can do amazing things. Your baby will look at your face. They turn towards your voice. They can suck on your breast or your clean finger. They can hold onto your finger.

Think about how new the world is for baby. Until now, they lived curled up in a warm, dark, watery place. They heard the beat of your heart and rush of your blood. Now the world has bright lights, sharp noises, cool air, and open space. Loud noises make baby jump. Bright lights make them blink. They feel things like cold and hunger for the first time. What a lot of change all at once!

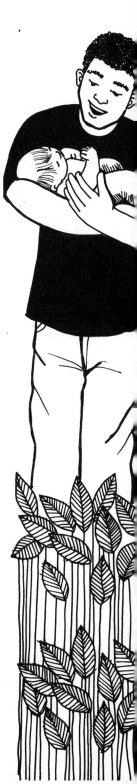

Babies start learning about the world as soon as they are born. Their brains grow and learn faster in the first three years than at any other time.

The most important people in your baby's world are you and the others who care for them. Your family will grow together by caring for this new baby.

A good start for the whole family

A baby grows best in a happy home. It is important for parents to try to listen to and support each other. You will need extra help in the first few months while your body heals and you spend time with the baby. A partner can also need help. Older children will need more attention and love at this time, too.

Your first days as a parent

Your main jobs now are to get to know your baby, make sure baby is fed, and help your body heal. (For more about your own recovery, see chapter 15.)

"I tell myself that feeding time is when I am not allowed to think about all the things I need to do. It helps me enjoy and look forward to it."

Take time to slow down and relax with baby. Get comfortable and have a snack while you feed baby.

Take naps or rest when your baby sleeps. Ask your partner, family, and friends to do cooking, shopping, and laundry. If you are tired from too many guests or phone calls, it is okay to say "not now." Ask them to call in a week or two.

You may feel like you don't know how to care for baby. This is a common feeling. You will learn as you go along.

Don't be shy. Ask for help. Nurses, breastfeeding consultants, and others can show you how to do things. But, you can also do things your way. You'll be surprised by how much you figure out for yourself.

Partners as parents

As a partner, you are a key part of the parent team. Your partner and baby both need you! You are very important in baby's life. You will learn your own ways of caring for your child.

The more time you spend with your baby, the more comfortable you will feel. Take time to touch, cuddle, and talk to your baby. They will learn quickly to know your voice, smell, and touch. Hold baby close and talk or sing in a high, happy voice. Take care of baby by yourself sometimes. The more you practice, the better you'll feel about comforting baby or changing diapers.

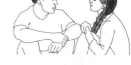

You and your partner will need teamwork to get things done around the house. Focus on the most important tasks, like laundry or shopping. Other things like vacuuming or lawn mowing can wait. Take time to rest, eat, and think about all that is going on. It's important to take care of yourself, too.

Watch out for moods that get worse

Feeling tired or having the baby blues is normal in the first few weeks after your baby is born. These feelings go away with rest, support from friends, and time. But sometimes these feelings get worse. Many parents feel extra sad, mad, or anxious and it doesn't go away. This is a sign of a problem. Watch out for each other. Learn more about what to watch for and how to get help in chapter 16.

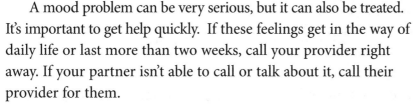

A mood problem can be very serious, but it can also be treated. It's important to get help quickly. If these feelings get in the way of daily life or last more than two weeks, call your provider right away. If your partner isn't able to call or talk about it, call their provider for them.

Older children at home

If you have other children, they may get tired of the new baby pretty quickly. The baby will take most of your time. This can make the other kids act needy or angry. This is normal. Here are some ways to help them:

◆ Spend some special time with each older child every day. Let them know you still love them just as much as before.

◆ Let siblings "help" you with baby. Diaper changes are great for this. They can bring you the wipes and a clean diaper. They can make silly faces or sing to baby to keep them calm. Older kids can hold baby for you while you cook or even feed them a bottle.

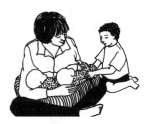

Always stay nearby when baby is with other kids. It's safest not to leave baby alone with children under 13 years old. Even

Big brother helping out.

then, some kids aren't ready to handle problems if something goes wrong.

Grandparents and other family members

It is good for babies to get to know their grandparents, aunts, uncles, and cousins. Some relatives may help care for your baby a lot.

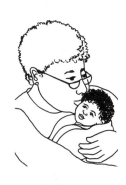

A visiting nurse, case worker, or baby's provider can help talk with your family, too.

Family can be a big help, but they may have old ideas of how to care for a baby. Many older relatives may not like newer advice like putting baby on their back for sleep. Tell them that baby's safety is important to you. Ask them to take a baby safety class and learn CPR. Give them this book to refresh what they know about baby care. Let them know you value their advice and want their support. But keep in mind that it's also okay to disagree with them.

Remember that you and your partner are the parents. You make the decisions about what is best for your baby. You've worked hard to learn and make choices for your family.

If you are a teen, you may need your family's help with baby. You will need to be able to talk to each other about how to care for baby. There will be many choices for you to make and it's really helpful if they agree. If they want to know why you want things a certain way, tell them. If they don't agree, ask them why. If you still can't agree, ask yourself if it's okay to do things different from each other. Often it is, like how you soothe or burp the baby. Sometimes it's not, like how to use the car seat correctly. Keep in mind that you all want what's best for baby.

Help with twins, triplets, or more babies

One baby is a lot of work. If you have twins or triplets (or more), you and your partner will need more help. Local groups for parents of twins can give you very useful advice and support. Look for Mothers of Twins or Multiples groups and other resources listed in chapter 17.

Understanding your new baby

Your newborn baby can't talk, but does try to let you know what they want. Watch what your baby does. You, your partner, and other caregivers will learn what baby's sounds and faces mean. This will help meet baby's needs. (Which also helps them cry less!)

How does baby act when sleeping?

- **When baby is in a deep sleep,** they breathe slowly and do not wake up easily. This is a good time to move baby, like from car seat to crib.

- **When baby is in a light sleep,** their breathing will be less regular. Their eyes may move under their lids. Their mouth may look like it's sucking. Their arms and legs may move. Baby wakes easily.

- **If baby starts to wake after sleeping only a short time,** wait a few minutes before picking them up. Put your hand on their chest and whisper "shh shh". Offer a pacifier. Baby may go back to sleep.

How does baby act when awake?

- **When your baby is waking up** they may need some quiet time before they are ready to eat or play. Talk softly, give gentle rubs, or calmly change their diaper.

- **When baby is awake and alert** they will look at you and listen to your voice. This is a good time to play. A newborn baby may only be able to do this for a minute or two at a time. When they look away or turn their head, it means they need to rest. (Eye contact is a lot of work!) This is a good time to calmly cuddle your baby.

- **If your baby is fussy,** they may need your help to calm down. Make sure you are calm first. Then hold baby close and rock them, or use a baby carrier to take them for a walk.

- **When baby is hungry,** they may stick their tongue out or make sucking sounds. They may turn toward you or suck on whatever they can reach. These are early hunger signs. Try to feed baby now, instead of after they start to cry.

- **When your baby is getting tired,** they may blink very slowly. Their arms and legs will slow down and jerk if startled. They may sigh or make soft sounds. This sleepy signs are a good time to put baby to sleep, before they start to cry.

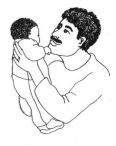

"I just wanted to play with baby when I got home. But they just kept crying more and more. I finally figured out that they were too tired to play and just needed cuddles at that time. Now we have play time before I leave in the morning."

Every baby is different

Each baby has their own personality early on. Some are very calm and quiet, watching what is going on around them. Others may be shy. Some are very active and easy to excite. Watch your baby to see what you notice.

Talking to your new baby

Your baby can hear the sounds around them as soon as they are born. They are getting ready to talk long before they know what words mean.

Hold baby close to your face while you talk softly. Talk slowly in a high, sing-song voice. You can use real words, not just "baby talk." Show baby a picture book and tell them about the pictures. Or just talk about the things you do all day. Soon baby will start making their own sounds ("coo" and later "da-da-da"). When your

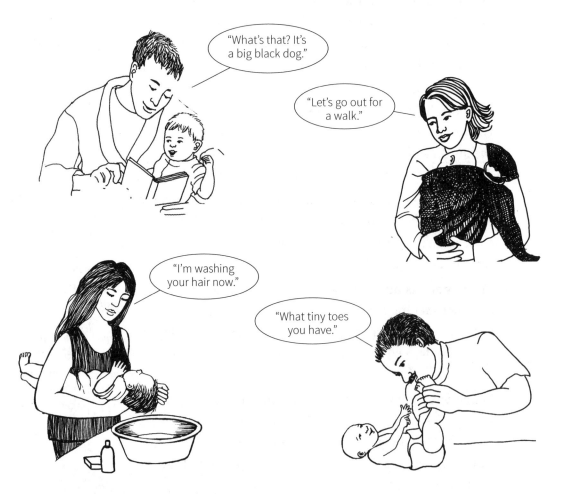

baby does this, it is good to make those same sounds back. This kind of "talking" back and forth helps their brain grow.

A baby can hear the sounds of all languages in the first six to nine months. If you or any family members speak other languages, it is good for your baby to hear those sounds now.

Playing with your new baby

Playing helps your baby connect with you and learn. When baby is alert, play with them by:

+ making faces at them. Hold baby 8 to 10 inches from your face. Open your mouth or stick your tongue out and wait a minute or two for them to react. If they make a face, do it back to them.

+ lifting them gently into the air or gently swinging them side to side.

+ singing short songs like "Twinkle, Twinkle Little Star."

+ gently touching baby's body. Slide your hands from the top of their head, gently squeeze their shoulders, stroke their arms. Pat their belly, stroke their legs, and squeeze their feet. Make up a rhyme or just tell them what you're doing.

+ shake a rattle or a bell. smack your lips, click your tongue, or whistle. see what baby does.

+ hold baby up to look in a mirror.

If your baby was born very early, they may not be ready to play until a bit after their due date. Before that time, they just need to see your face, hear your voice, and feel your touch.

Always play gently – Never, never shake a baby!

Make sure that anyone who plays with your baby always is very gentle. New babies have very large, heavy heads and their necks are weak. It's important to always support their head and neck. Especially when bouncing or moving around a lot. Rough play or strong jerking movements can cause serious brain injury.

Tummy time for baby

"My baby loved lying on a quilt with big, bright red and yellow ladybugs on it. They would lift their head to look."

It is important for baby to have some time on their tummy every day. This helps strengthen their neck and arm muscles. They will practice lifting and moving their head. Soon they will start turning it from side to side. Then they will start pushing up with their arms and legs.

Play with your baby on their tummy for a few minutes two or three times a day.

- Let them lie on your chest while you lie or sit reclined.
- Lay them on a clean cloth on the floor. Try a play mat or a quilt with bright colors. Switch which way baby's head is turned after a bit.
- Let them lie on a knit blanket with little lumps in it so they can feel rough textures. They learn a lot by touching.
- Sit or lie down next to them so they can see your face or hands. Talk or sing, or pat their back. Pat the blanket in front of them or hold out a colorful toy.
- Wear them in a baby carrier for walks sometimes so you can be close, talk, and see their face.

Sitting up in a play seat, swing, or car seat

The safest way for baby to spend time is lying flat on their back or being held. Their neck isn't strong enough to hold their head up for very long. When baby's head flops forward, it makes it hard for them to breathe well. Baby's airway is clearest when their chin bone is up off of their chest.

If baby's head flops down chin to chest when you sit them up, wait a while and do more tummy time. If you do use a swing or play seat, check their chin and buckle the safety straps. Keep baby where you can see them.

Any time your baby is in their car seat, keep them as reclined as their seat allows, with their straps buckled and snug. (Even if they're not in the car!)

Preventing a flat spot on baby's head

Some babies start to get flat areas on the back of their heads. This can happen if they spend a lot of time lying on their back. This also can come from sitting for long times in a baby seat, car seat, or swing.

If you think your baby might be getting a flat spot, ask about it at your baby's next checkup.

Use the tips below to help baby's head stay round as it grows. Ways to prevent a flat spot:

- Switch ends of the crib often to keep baby from always lying with their head on the same side.
- Use tummy time when baby is awake. Move toys or your face from side to side to get baby to turn their head.
- Use a baby seat or swing only for short times.
- Use the car seat for travel, not as a place to sleep, eat, or play at home.
- Use a baby carrier sometimes instead of a stroller.

How your baby develops

Watch how your new baby changes. Do they show signs that they can see and hear? Are they learning new things? This is development. Every baby has four kinds of development.

1. Learning to relate to people (like smiling) and trust them (getting comfort from a parent)
2. Physical changes (like rolling over, picking up things with fingers)
3. Thinking and learning (like knowing the faces of people they see often, looking at colors)
4. Language (like showing what they want with sounds or signs long before they can talk)

Baby's development and you

Babies grow best when they feel safe and loved. Every baby's development is closely tied to what parents do, feel, and say. Babies learn trust when parents feed them when they are hungry, and comfort them when they are upset. This helps baby know that parents will take care of them. It makes them feel safe.

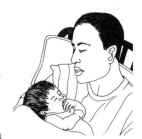

Every new parent needs to learn to respond to their child in a caring way. If you have a hard time cuddling, holding, or feeding

Changes as babies grow and learn

Watch for these signs of change

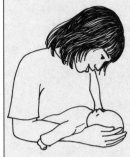

1 week

Most newborns:

- Like to look at a face 8 to 12 inches away
- Follow your face when you move side to side
- React to sounds (by blinking, startling, crying)

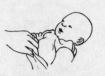

1 month

At 1 month, most babies:

- Respond to your face and voice
- Turn their head from side to side while on tummy
- Put their hands in their mouths
- Stop crying if picked up and cuddled

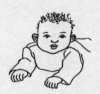

2 months

At 2–3 months, most babies:

- Smile when you smile at them
- Turn their head toward sounds
- Make soft cooing sounds
- Lift their head while lying on tummy
- Start to hold up their head when upright
- Calm themselves down some of the time

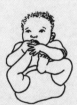

5 months

At 4–5 months, most babies:

- Start to roll over from tummy to back
- Smile, laugh, and babble
- Reach for, hold, and put toes in mouth
- Follow a moving toy back and forth with their eyes

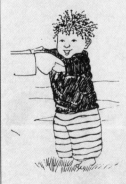

7 months

At 6–7 months, most babies:

- Like seeing faces they know, get nervous with strangers
- Smile at themselves in the mirror, know their own name
- Roll both ways, sit up, and stand with support
- Pass toys from one hand to the other

Check out resources in chapter 17.

baby, talk to your provider. Sometimes it's hard to stay calm when baby is very needy. They may have tips or be able to help you find support.

These early months of baby's life are so important. If you feel depressed, be sure to get help for yourself quickly. Family stress about money or other things can make it hard to give your energy to your baby. Again, tell someone you trust, so you can get help. (See chapter 16.)

Baby's leaps in learning

One of the most exciting things about parenting is watching as baby learns. From week to week, you'll see sudden changes. Baby will be really fussy for a few days and then suddenly do something new. This is a "leap" in learning. The first leap usually happens at about four to five weeks and the next at eight to nine weeks. It's common for baby to be really tired and fussy right before each leap. But they calm down soon after their new skill comes out.

Around five weeks, your baby may start smiling and looking at things longer. At nine weeks, you may see them playing with their hands or watching a toy move back and forth.

There will be lots more leaps as baby grows. Whenever they are fussy for a few days without any reason you can find, watch for a new skill!

Watching for delays in development

If you are worried about how well your baby is learning, tell their provider. Each baby learns at their own speed, but every baby should keep developing. You know your baby best. If you think they are learning too slowly, get help soon. The earlier, the better.

Keep track of baby's changes, new skills, and things that worry you. If you think they aren't doing what they should be, ask for a developmental screening. A provider will check your baby's growth and skills and compare them to what most babies their age can do. If there are any concerns, they will talk to you about what you can do to help.

See chapter 17 for resources about baby's development.

Signs that baby is ready to sleep

◆ They look away and do not want to play.

◆ They yawn, rub their eyes, and make soft, fussy noises.

◆ Their eyes keep closing.

Getting baby to sleep

Sleep is good for babies. It's also good for parents! But some babies sleep less than others. It can be very hard if yours is one who likes to stay awake.

Getting baby to go to sleep is not always easy. You will hear many ideas about how to do it. There is no one right way for all babies. Try different things to see what works for you and your baby.

It may seem easiest to let your baby fall asleep during feeding. However, this can become tricky if they get used to falling asleep in your arms or at your breast. It can be hard to change that habit later.

Make a bedtime routine that is the same each night. Read books, play soft music, and rock them to calm down. Start getting ready for bed before they seem ready to sleep. If you wait until baby is fussy, it may mean they are too tired to calm down and fall asleep.

When you see the sleepy signs, lay baby gently on their back in their bed. Keep the room quiet and dark. Gently rub or pat baby's tummy, whispering "shhh . . . shhh . . . shhh." Look away or close your eyes. Baby may fuss at first, but learning to calm down is part of their development.

If baby's sleep becomes a problem for you, talk with their provider. And remember, like all things with babies, their sleep will change as they grow.

When your baby cries

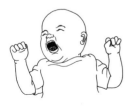

All babies cry. It is normal. It is how they ask for help or tell you that you haven't understood what they wanted. However, crying can make parents feel stressed, worried, or even mad.

As baby gets older, they will have different cries for when they are hungry, tired, wet, lonely, uncomfortable, bored, or sick. You will learn what they are trying to tell you. Even if you don't know why they are crying, you can still try to comfort them. You can't spoil a baby by holding them when they cry.

Things that usually calm a crying baby

- Make sure your baby does not have a fever or other signs of illness (chapter 15).
- Change their diaper. Try to burp them.
- If it's been more than an hour since they ate, offer them milk. If they don't want it, offer a clean finger or pacifier for comfort sucking.
- Try swaddling them. If they are already swaddled, take their arms out so they can use their hands.
- Hold them on their tummy and rock or sway.
- Put them in a carrier and take a walk inside or outside.
- Make soothing sounds like "shhh, shhh, shhh," over and over again. Some babies like soft singing or dull background noise like the sound of a fan or dryer.
- If they've been awake for a while, they could be overtired. See if they'll fall asleep in their crib while you gently pat them or sing.
- All babies cry some throughout the day. Most crying can be soothed. But if your baby cries often or for very long periods of time, and can't be soothed, talk to their provider. They can help make sure there's nothing serious going on.

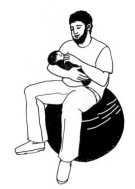

Gentle bouncing can be very soothing for a crying baby.

When the crying won't stop

Most babies have a time of day or night when they are very fussy. For some babies, this might just be needing to be held for comfort. But for others, it means crying so hard they gasp for air, no matter what you do to soothe them. This fussy time is common in the first few months. It's worst around two months and mostly gone after four months.

If they don't have signs of sickness, check their comfort. Are they cold, hot, hungry, sleepy, or needing a burp or diaper change? If not, they are likely just fine. Their brain is growing a lot at this time and can get sort of stuck on crying for a bit. But just because it's normal, doesn't mean it's not really hard on you.

"My mom said it's colic, but the doctor said it's not. Nothing's wrong with my baby's body. They just need to cry a lot right now. But it's really hard for me."

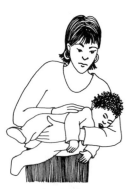

A crying baby may like to be held with your arm under their tummy.

Try these tips for soothing:

- **Music:** Play soft music. Sing or hum so they hear your voice.

- **Movement:** Hold baby and dance, sway, rock, or bounce gently.

- **Cuddle:** Put baby in a carrier so they're close and facing you. Or, take shirts off and snuggle skin to skin with a blanket wrapped around you both.

- **Change things up:** If you are warm inside, take baby outside where it's cold. If it's quiet, turn on some music. If it's bright, go somewhere dark.

- **Get up and go:** Take baby for a walk if you need a bit of space. Or, go for a car ride together.

If these things don't work, you haven't failed and baby is okay. Let someone else take a turn. Or start over with the basics, like feeding and a diaper change. It can be very hard, but sometimes you may have to just wait it out.

Get help for yourself when your baby keeps crying

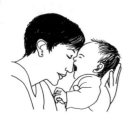

Crying is very hard on the person taking care of baby. When it won't stop, it is very stressful for anyone. You might worry that something is wrong with you or the baby. You might feel like crying, yelling, or shaking.

All of these are signs that you need to take a time out, for your sake and for the baby's. Make a plan for what to do when you have tried everything, baby is still crying, and you are getting upset.

A plan might look like this:

1. Swaddle baby and put them in a safe place like their crib and leave the room. Baby will be okay crying there for a few minutes.

2. Take a few deep breaths and put on some music so you can't really hear the crying. Close your eyes.

3. Remind yourself that baby isn't choosing to cry. They're not trying to make you mad or hurt you.

4. Tell yourself you are not doing anything wrong. Call a friend who you can tell how frustrated you feel.

5. Put a cool cloth on your face or drink a glass of water. Avoid alcohol or drugs.

6. Remember, this hard time will get better when baby gets a little older.

7. Once you're calm, go back to baby and try again.

It can be hard to stay calm when baby cries a lot.

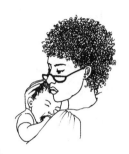

You must take care of yourself, too. Ask someone you trust to take care of baby sometimes. Make sure it's someone you know won't get upset if baby cries. Take time to relax or get things done.

NEVER shake your baby!

It's important to put baby down in a safe place and go into the next room if you feel really upset. Have a drink of water. Call a friend to give you a break. Or call a hotline to talk.

See chapter 17 for a list of places that can help.

Shaking, hitting, dropping, or throwing a baby can badly hurt their brain. This is called **shaken baby syndrome** or **abusive head trauma**, and it can't be undone. Most of these brain injuries happen when a baby won't stop crying and the adult doesn't put baby down in time. **If you think your baby has been shaken, call 911.**

If you need help now, call or text 988 or visit *988lifeline.org* **to chat.**

Tips for partners

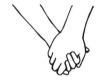

◆ Hold your baby. Smile and talk to them. Make faces and wait for them to react. Read or point at pictures in a book. Baby will play with toys when they're a bit older. Right now, they will love just watching you and being with you.

◆ Spend time with your partner. You're a family now. It's important to show that you value and respect your partner as a parent. It is also good for your baby to see that you care for each other.

◆ Be patient. This can be a very hard time for you, too. Talk with a friend or counselor.

◆ If your baby cries non-stop for part of the day, remember it will pass. This is a time when teamwork is most important for you and your partner.

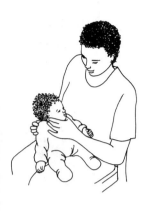

- Take turns caring for baby. You will find your own ways to feed or burp your baby, calm their cries, or get them to sleep. It is good for you and baby to have time together. It's also good for your partner to get a break.

- Learn how to give baby a bath. Make it fun with silly faces and songs. After bath, give baby a gentle massage with olive oil.

- Watch out for signs of mood problems. Be honest and kind with your partner. Speak up if you are worried. These illnesses can happen to partners, too. Talk to someone about your feelings. Ask for help when you need it.

Chapter 14

Keeping Your Baby Safe

It's scary to think about anything happening to your new baby. Learn how to protect them now. This means you can worry less. For healthy babies, the biggest dangers in the first year are:

- SIDS (Sudden Infant Death Syndrome).
- Suffocation during sleep.
- Car crashes.
- Falls.

It is hard to believe that sleeping or riding in a car could hurt your baby. They are things we all do every day. Most of the time, nothing bad happens. But there is always a risk of something very serious. Every parent—and every other caregiver—needs to learn how to keep babies safe.

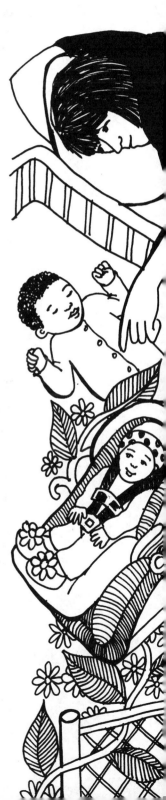

Look in this chapter for:

How can sleep be dangerous?

Sleep is good for babies, as long as they're on their back in a safe space. In the US, more than 3,000 babies die from sleep-related deaths each year. Most of these deaths are from unknown causes or Sudden Infant Death Syndrome (SIDS). The rest are caused by baby's airway being blocked by something (suffocation or strangulation). Even if the cause of death isn't known, it is known that:

- most young babies (birth to 3 months) were in bed with another person.

- most older babies (4 to 12 months) had soft things in bed with them (pillows, blankets, stuffed animals, etc.).

Sudden infant death syndrome (SIDS)

When a baby (12 months or younger) dies in their sleep area with no known cause of death, it may be called a SIDS death. It is most common in babies less than 6 months old. It's no one's fault when a baby dies of SIDS. No one knows for sure what causes it, so no one can say how to prevent it. There are ways we can make it less likely, though. (See below.)

Suffocation and strangulation

A baby **suffocates** when they can't breathe because something blocked their mouth and nose. This can happen if someone rolls on top of baby. It can also happen if baby rolls over into a pillow or has a blanket over their face. Babies do not have the strength or skill to move their head if they get stuck.

A baby is **strangled** when they can't breathe due to something tight around their neck. This can happen with a baby monitor cord or the edge of a crib bumper. Babies move a lot in their sleep and can get tangled up easily.

How can I keep baby safe while they sleep?

There are many ways to protect baby while they sleep. Two of the biggest things are to make sure:

- baby's sleep space is as safe as possible.
- baby is put to sleep lying flat on their back.

Studies show that the couch is the most dangerous place for a baby to sleep.

A safe sleep space

Baby is safest on a firm, flat baby bed that follows safety standards (see chapter 6). This could be a crib, play yard*, or bassinet. If you can't get a baby bed, do the best you can. You could use a strong box or laundry basket placed on the floor.

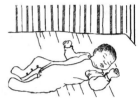

A safe sleep space has:

- a firm, flat surface with no way for baby to fall off.
- a mattress that fits the baby bed with no gaps at the edges where baby's head could get stuck.
- no blankets, pillows, or soft toys.
- no padded bumper or sleep positioner.

***Play yard:**
A pop-up baby bed with mesh sides, often called a "pack'n'play." Make sure it meets safety standards. Some "co-sleepers" are play yards that meet safety standards, but many are not.

Dangerous places for baby to sleep

- On a sofa, couch, chair, or waterbed
- In a bed with an adult, another child, or a pet
- With an adult who has been using alcohol or drugs. (Some medicines can make you sleepy enough to roll over onto your baby.)
- In other baby gear, like swings, bouncers, rockers, or car seats (except when driving). Always buckle baby in and stay where you can see them.

Think it through before putting your baby to sleep anywhere other than a baby bed. What are the risks? How can I make it as safe as possible?

On their back to sleep

Put your baby on their back to sleep, every time they sleep, from day one. The sooner you start, the safer baby will be. They may not like it at first, but they'll learn to sleep that way with some help. Tummy or side sleeping is risky for young babies.

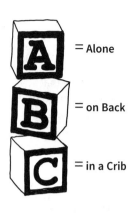

= Alone

= on Back

= in a Crib

Won't baby choke?

Most babies are less likely to choke on their spit up if they are flat on their back. Babies are more likely to choke if they are more upright.

What if my baby rolls over?

If your very young baby rolls onto their tummy while they sleep, you can roll them back over. Being on a soft surface that is not all the way flat can make baby roll.

After a few months, if your baby has learned how to roll back and forth between back and tummy, you can let them sleep that way. But you should still put baby down on their back and let them roll on their own if they want. Also be sure baby's sleep area is clear of any soft things or cords.

Once baby can roll, stop swaddling or do it with arms out.

Some preemies or sick babies may be on their tummies in the hospital. They have lots of people and machines making sure they're safe. Most babies will be switched to sleeping on their back before they go home. Ask their provider if there is a medical reasons to sleep on their tummy at home. If not, baby is safest on their back.

"My new baby kept flipping over. When I stopped swaddling, they stayed on their back!"

More important safe sleep tips

- ◆ Breastfeed your baby or feed them breast milk.
- ◆ Make sure there's no smoke (or e-cigarette vapor) near baby before or after they are born. No smoking in the house or the car.
- ◆ Keep your baby's bed in the same room where you sleep. It is safest to share a room, not a bed.
- ◆ Dress baby in pajamas that will keep them warm, but not hot. If they are swaddled, they may just need a onesie underneath. If baby wakes up sweaty or with a red face they were too hot. Keep your heater set below 73°F (22.8°C).
- ◆ Give your baby a pacifier as they fall asleep. Offer it for sleep, even if they don't want it while awake. See chapter 12 for more on pacifiers.

"I was worried my baby's head would get flat sleeping on their back, but the doctor said lots of tummy time when baby's awake will prevent that."

- Vaccinate your baby on time.
- Keep all cords 3 feet or more away from baby's bed. Cords on window blinds and monitors can be deadly.

Even if you can't do **all** of these things, you're still helping your baby be safer.

Be careful with bed-sharing

The safest way for baby to sleep is in their own bed in your room. Use a bassinet, play yard, or crib next to your bed. There should be nothing above baby. The side of baby's bed should be higher than yours so nothing can fall on baby. If it isn't, move baby's bed an arm's reach away from yours. If baby falls asleep with you, move them to their own bed.

A baby who sleeps in bed with adults or other kids is more likely to suffocate. This can happen if someone rolls onto baby or if baby gets stuck against the bed, wall, or furniture. But a lot of babies end up sleeping with their parents. It may seem like the only way to get any sleep. Or, there may not be space for a crib in the room.

It's very important to think about safety before you bring baby into bed with you, even just once. Your pillows, blankets, and even your long hair can be dangerous.

If baby does end up in your bed, try to make it safer. This can be hard. Make sure:

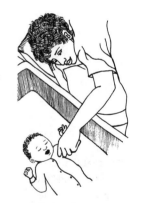

Baby's crib next to parents' bed—a safe place to sleep.

- baby sleeps on their back, not swaddled, and is not too warm.
- there are no pillows or heavy blankets on or nearby.
- the mattress is very firm.
- there is no space around the bed where baby's head could get stuck.
- baby cannot fall off of the bed.
- everyone in the bed is sober. no drugs, alcohol, or medicines that make them sleep really deeply.
- baby does not sleep between two people.
- baby does not have other health problems. healthy, full-term babies may be safer than others.

Teach your baby's caregivers about sleep safety

Make sure all people who care for your baby know to always put baby on their back for sleep. When a baby is used to sleeping on their back, SIDS may be even more likely if they sleep on their tummy just once. Explain why soft things like blankets can be dangerous. Even when others don't agree, you get to make the rules about keeping your baby safe.

Car seat safety

Everyone in the car should be buckled up for every ride, even if it's short. Your baby must ride in a car seat that fits. Car seats are very good at saving lives. If baby's car seat is the right size and you learn how to use it right, your baby will be the safest person in the car. Car seat use is the same if baby is in a minivan, SUV, pickup truck, or taxi.

If you often take your baby in a school bus or transit bus, see page 240. Safety will be different if there are no seat belts.

Rear facing is safest

All babies and toddlers should ride rear-facing (facing the back of the car) as long as possible. Riding rear-facing is safest. This is because the back of the car seat protects baby's head, neck, and back from being thrown forward. Injuries are worst to these parts of the body. Even in very bad crashes, kids riding rear-facing are usually not hurt.

Car seat limits: "Too tall" and "too heavy" means they have reached the limits for that car seat. Check your seat's labels or manual for its rear-facing limits.

Keep baby riding rear-facing until they are too tall or too heavy for their car seat*. Most convertible car seats will fit most kids rear-facing until they are 2 to 4 years old.

Choosing the "best" car seat

There are a lot of car seats out there! It can be very hard to choose. There is not one best brand. The best car seat is the one that:

+ has low harness (shoulder) slots to fit a new baby.
+ is labeled for use by babies as small as five pounds.
+ fits your car's back seat and can be buckled in tightly.
+ is easy to use properly on every car ride.

See chapter 6 for how to choose the best car seat for you. Be sure to try it in your car before you buy it.

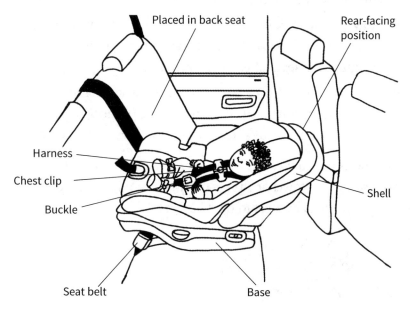

A rear-facing car seat

Installing the car seat

Use the middle seating position in the back seat if the car seat can be installed tightly there. If you are carrying other children or if it doesn't fit there, move it to the side.

Read the car seat booklet. It tells you what you need to know about using the car seat. Read about how to buckle it to the car and baby into the seat.

Read your car's owner's manual. Read the part that talks about installing car seats. (Car seats may be called "child restraint systems.") See if your car has LATCH* (sometimes called **ISOFIX**). If your car has LATCH, find out where and how you can use it. Also read how to use the seat belts to attach the car seat.

*LATCH: A way of buckling a car seat into a car instead of using a seat belt. LATCH uses special parts in the car and on the car seat. (It is sometimes called **ISOFIX**.)

- Where do you want baby to ride? If you want to put them in the middle of the back seat, you may need to use the seat belt. Most cars don't allow LATCH use there.

- Can you use LATCH? To use it, both the car and the car seat must have special parts that connect together. LATCH

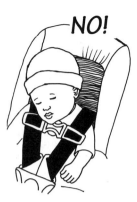

NO!

If baby's head flops forward, adjust the seat to tip back a bit more.

may not be usable in every seat in the car. It can only be used until your child reaches a certain weight. Once your child is too heavy, use the seat belt.

◆ How do you lock the seat belts? There are a few kinds of seat belts. Each has a different way of being tightened around a car seat. Check the car manual.

◆ How far should the car seat be tipped back (reclined)? Follow the recline indicator on the side of most seats. Make sure your baby's head doesn't fall forward (picture).

Most seats have a way to change the recline angle. If yours doesn't, use a rolled towel or a piece of a foam "pool noodle" under the car seat by the baby's feet to tilt it back a bit.

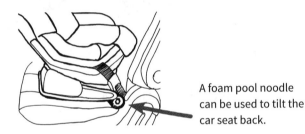

A foam pool noodle can be used to tilt the car seat back.

Install the car seat tightly with the car's seat belt or LATCH. To test if it is tight, push and pull on the car seat base. The seat shouldn't move more than one inch side to side or front to back.

Air bags and babies

Never place your baby in the front seat with an air bag unless the air bag has been turned off. A baby can die if the front passenger air bag inflates. Put the car seat in front only if your car or truck has no back seat, or a very small one.

If the only place for baby to ride is in front, you must make sure the air bag is turned off. Read about it in the car manual. There will be either an air bag sensor* or a switch to turn the air bag off and on. Sensors turn the air bag off automatically. If there is a switch, you must turn off the air bag while a baby or child is riding in front. The air bag light on the dashboard tells you if the air bag is off or on. (Turn it on again when adults and teens are riding there.)

If you have a really old car and aren't sure it has a front passenger air bag, look for a warning label on the sun visor. The car owner's manual will have details about air bags if it has them.

*Sensor:
An electronic device that automatically turns off the air bag when a small child is riding in the front seat. The owner's manual will tell if the car has sensors.

Buckling your baby into the car seat

1. The crotch strap must go between baby's legs.

2. Shoulder straps should come out of the seat at baby's shoulder or a bit lower. It is not safe for them to be above baby's shoulders.

3. The harness must be snug. To test it, pinch the strap between your fingers (see picture). If you can pinch any slack, it is not snug enough.

4. Put the chest clip so it points to your baby's armpits.

Pinch the strap to see if it is too loose. This one needs to be tightened.

Helpful car seat tips

♦ Many car seats come with pads. (Some even have pads under the cover!) If yours did, check the manual to see how and when to use them. If your baby still flops forward, check to see if it's okay to take the pads out.

♦ **Do not** use any pads, covers, or other things that did not come with your car seat. Many can be dangerous in a crash. Others can be harmful any time baby sits in the car seat.

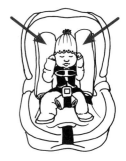

♦ Dress baby in clothes that fit well and leave their legs free. Pants, pajamas, and onesies leave room to safely use the crotch buckle. Avoid dresses, gowns, and tutu skirts. Do not swaddle baby before you buckle and tighten the straps.

If there are no pads and baby is slumping:
♦ buckle and tighten baby's straps.
♦ chest clip to armpit level.
♦ place snugly rolled blankets in the gap on each side of baby.
♦ **do not** add any padding under, above, or behind baby.

♦ In cold weather, put your baby in thin fleece or wool pants or pajamas. Do not use a padded snowsuit or bunting. After baby's buckled in and the straps are snug, you can cover baby's lap with a blanket. Tuck it around their arms and legs. Don't forget to take blankets off as the car warms up so baby doesn't get too warm.

Getting help with using your car seat

Car seats can be confusing. Most car seats are used wrong in some ways. Have your car seat checked by a certified Child Passenger Safety Technician. Checkups are very helpful and they are usually free.

See chapter 17 for how to find a car seat check near you.

"My friend gave me a puffy snowsuit. It was so thick I couldn't get the car seat harness tight. So I only use it in the stroller."

Car beds for babies with breathing problems

Some babies have medical problems and need to lie flat. These babies may have to ride in a special car bed. Babies who are born very early may breathe better flat on their back for a few weeks. Other babies may need to ride lying down for longer because of health issues. If your baby needs a car bed, ask your nurse or Child Passenger Safety Technician to help you get one.

This car bed is mainly for preemies.

All preemies born before 37 weeks should be tested sitting in their car seat before leaving the hospital. This is to make sure baby can breathe well sitting up. If the baby has any trouble breathing, they should ride lying flat for a few weeks. (Baby also should not sit in a swing or baby seat at home until they are older.)

Car seats in taxis and school or transit buses

Use a car seat in any vehicle with seat belts, like a taxi. Do it the same way as you do in a regular car.

If you are a teen, you may take your baby with you in a school bus. In some places buses have seat belts. You may be able to use a small rear-facing car seat. Ask your driver if the district provides car seats.

In buses (or trains) without seat belts, there's no really safe way to carry baby. Sit with baby in a seat that faces forward, not the side of the bus. A car seat with a handle might give some protection even if it's not buckled in. Always use baby's harness in the seat. You could wear baby in a carrier. That would allow your hands to be free for holding on.

Never leave baby alone in a car!

Babies die every year from being left alone in a parked car. A parked car can turn into an oven quickly. Even if it's not hot outside, the car can get really hot in just a few minutes. Cracking a window or parking in the shade doesn't help.

Some babies are left in the car to nap. Others get left behind when their adult's quick stop takes longer than planned.

Sometimes babies are forgotten in the car by tired or stressed parents or other caregivers. Here are ways to prevent leaving baby in the car.

◆ Make a habit of putting your bag or backpack on the floor of the back seat. This will make you look in back when you get out.

◆ If your baby goes to child care, ask the caregiver to call if baby isn't there by a certain time.

Using other gear safely

Using a cloth baby carrier

When you wear your baby in a carrier or sling, remember these safety tips, called TICKS:

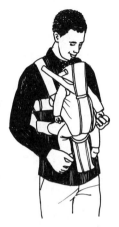

T—Tight, hugging baby to your body

I—In view, where you can see baby's face easily

C—Close enough to kiss the top of baby's head

K—Keep baby's neck straight, not flopped forward or back

S—Support baby's back so they're not curled up or chin to chest.

Use a carrier that has head support and keeps baby up high on your chest.

Learn how to put baby into your carrier with a friend helping to make sure baby doesn't fall. Or, try it sitting on your bed, just in case. After you get baby in, look in a mirror and go through the TICKS checklist above. Make sure to read all instructions for your carrier.

If you have a used carrier, check it for recalls. Make sure it is in good shape with no holes, tears, or loose threads.

See chapter 17 for where to learn more about wearing your baby.

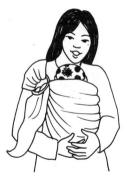

Keep baby upright in a sling.

Secondhand baby gear

Using gently used baby gear can save a lot of money. Avoid used car seats unless you know it hasn't been in a crash (chapter 6). For car seats and other gear, make sure you have the instructions so you can use it correctly. Check to see that all of the parts are there and put together well. Look to see if it has been recalled.

Stay away from old or recalled gear

There are many used baby seats out there that are not safe to use. Old, plastic carriers may look like a car seat but are very light and have thin straps or plastic buckles. A recalled baby rocker may look as safe as a bouncy seat. These old products are dangerous and should be taken apart and thrown away.

Learn what to do in an emergency

Plan ahead for when disaster strikes. What would you do if there was a fire in your home? Or if the power went out for a long time? Chapter 17 has resources to help you make a safety plan for your new family. Below are some basics.

Have a first aid kit

Keep a well-stocked first aid kit in your home. Keep it where you can get to it easily. It should have bandages, wound cleaner, antibacterial ointment, and tweezers. Infant acetaminophen (like Tylenol) and a digital thermometer should be added for baby. You may want to add things like eye drops, allergy medicine, and instant cold packs.

If you have a car, keep another first aid kit in there. Add things that would help if you were stuck in your car: food, water, formula, blankets, and diapers.

Learn CPR and choking rescue

Babies put everything in their mouths. Anything that fits in a toilet paper tube is small enough to choke on. Infant choking rescue is easy to learn and can save a life.

Cardiopulmonary resuscitation (CPR) is how you help someone who has stopped breathing and won't wake up. It keeps blood and oxygen moving through their body while you wait for help. It's very unlikely that you'd need to do CPR on your baby. But it's important to know how, just in case.

Find a class that teaches infant choking rescue and CPR. Make sure they have manikins you can practice on. Schools, fire stations, and community centers often have free classes. Learn more in the safety section of chapter 17.

Other ways to keep baby safe

Start baby proofing your home before baby is on the move. Making your home safer now means you can worry less later. Even simple changes can help keep baby safe.

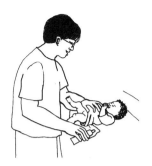

Keep one hand on baby.

Preventing falls

Babies are often wiggly and hard to hold onto. When you are busy or tired, it is easy to drop baby.

Try not to do too many things at once while holding baby. Use a carrier to wear baby when you need a free hand. (Make sure you use the carrier right, page 241.) If you have a lot to carry, put things in a backpack. If you have tasks to do, put baby in a safe place until you are done. Safe places for baby would be:

+ a crib or play yard.
+ a clear space on a clean floor.

A wiggly baby can slip off a bed or table. When you change, bathe, or dress your baby, always keep one hand on their body. Have everything you need where you can reach it before you start.

Other things you can do to keep baby safe from falls:

+ Never leave baby alone on a chair, table, bed, or counter, even for a second.
+ Always buckle safety straps on baby gear.
+ If baby is in a car seat or bouncy seat, don't put it on top of anything tall. Keep it on the floor.
+ Don't put baby's car seat on top of a shopping cart. If you do bring baby's seat into the store, put it in the big part of the cart. Wearing your baby leaves your hands free and keeps baby safe.
+ Put strong baby gates at the top and bottom of the stairs before baby learns to crawl. Keep them closed. Make sure the gate is made for use on stairs. Some are not strong enough. Get a gate you can open with one hand.
+ Don't put cribs or other furniture near windows. Use window locks to keep windows from opening more than 4 inches. That keeps a baby from falling out.

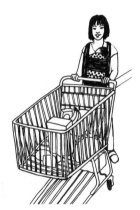

Shopping is a great time to wear your baby.

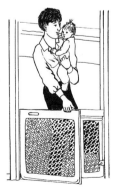

Use a gate you can open with one hand.

Preventing burns

Your baby's skin is very thin and can burn easily. Here are ways to prevent burns:

* **Bath temperature:** Make sure the bath water is just barely warm. Test it with your elbow. Turn down the temperature of your hot water heater to 120°F or 48.9°C.

* **Hot things around the house:** A curling iron, hot pan, or iron can fall on and burn a baby. Push them to the back of counters and put away cords where baby can't reach them.

* **Hot liquids:** Don't hold a hot drink or eat hot soup while you hold your baby. They could reach for it or bump it so it spills. Don't use the stove or microwave while holding baby, even in a carrier. Try to eat, drink, and cook while baby is playing or sleeping.

* **Things heated by the sun:** Things sitting in the sun can get too hot for baby's skin. Cover baby's car seat when it's left in the car. Always touch benches or swings before putting baby on them when you're out and about.

* **Sunburn:** When you are out in the sun, keep baby in the shade. Put them in a sun hat and clothes that cover their arms and legs. Use sunscreen on hands, feet, or other parts that show. See chapter 11 to learn more.

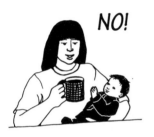

NO!

Don't drink hot liquids with baby in your lap.

Fire prevention – Smoke alarms

Smoke alarms can save your whole family from a house fire. Make sure you have at least one on each floor of your home. They are especially needed outside the bedrooms.

Carbon monoxide (CO) detectors can save your family from gas poisoning. CO is a deadly gas that you can't see or smell. CO detectors are needed if you have a gas stove or furnace, oil heat, or any kind of fireplace. Put one on each level of your home. If you can, put them below waist height.

Test all alarms often. Change the batteries at least once a year or put in 10-year batteries. Pick a day you will remember each year, like the day you turn the clocks ahead in spring.

Dangers as babies learn to crawl and climb

As your baby learns to crawl, stand, and climb, they are more likely to fall. Put gates at the top and bottom of stairs. Crawl through the house to see what baby could get into. Keep risky things where baby can't see or reach them. Lock up things that could be deadly.

- **Poisons and medicines:** Put all of your cleaners in a high cabinet and put a lock on it. Do the same with all of your medicines and vitamins. **Put Poison Control's phone number by all of your phones: 1-800-222-1222.**

- **Sharp things:** Keep knives and scissors out of reach.

- **Electric sockets and cords:** Put covers on electric outlets and put cords out of sight and reach. Tie up cords of curtains and window shades.

- **Heaters:** Put baby gates around the fireplace, wood stove, and heaters.

- **Guns:** Lock guns or other weapons in a gun safe.

Having dangerous things put out of reach or locked up makes caring for baby easier. It's more fun than saying "no" and taking things away all the time.

Babies will put anything in their mouths to learn about them. Sweep or vacuum the floor often. If you have pets, make sure their litter boxes, food, and water dishes are kept away from baby.

Babies like to pull themselves up when learning to walk. Some start climbing very early. Heavy things can tip over onto a baby. Bolt tall furniture like book shelves and dressers to the wall. Attach your TV to the wall so it can't fall.

No place is ever completely babyproof. As baby grows, watch out for new risks around the house and yard. Make sure that other homes where your baby spends time are also babyproofed. When you visit other places, watch baby closely just in case things are not as safe there.

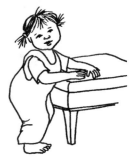

Soon your baby will be able get into things that you thought were out of reach.

Tips for partners

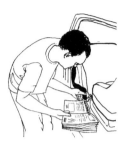

Use the vehicle and car seat manuals to use baby's car seat right.

- Have baby sleep in their own bed in your room. Talk to your partner about how you can help at night.
- Learn how to use your baby's car seat right: rear-facing with a snug harness. Make sure to follow the directions. Go to a car seat checkup with your partner.
- Learn the pinch test for car seat harness tightness. If you can squeeze a fold in the strap, it's too loose.
- Help with babyproofing. Make sure to close gates at the top and bottom of the stairs.
- Put all small things up high. Coins, keys, batteries, and other small things are dangerous for baby.
- Help keep the floors clean.
- Got your hands full? Wear baby in a carrier.

Chapter 15

Keeping Your Baby Healthy

Good health care is more than what your baby's doctor or nurse does. You, your partner, and baby's provider are a team. As the leader of this team, you will:

1. take baby for all of their checkups.
2. make sure baby gets vaccines on time.
3. learn to tell if baby is sick and when to call their provider.
4. learn how to take care of baby when they are sick.
5. give baby a safe home and do what you can to keep baby healthy.

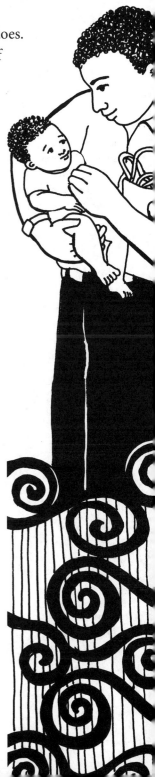

Look in this chapter for:

Tips for baby's health

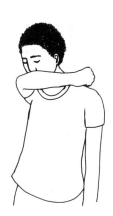

Cough into your arm or sleeve. This prevents hands from getting covered with germs and passing them on.

- Breastfeed your baby so they get antibodies from you to fight germs.
- Wash your hands often and make sure others do, too. If you can't wash, use hand sanitizer.
- Keep baby away from people who are smoking. Ask people who smoke to do it outside and wash their hands and change their clothes afterwards.
- If you cough or sneeze, cover your nose and mouth with your sleeve or arm, not your hand.
- Keep your baby away from people who have colds, coughs, fevers, or other sickness. They may not seem very sick. But they could spread germs that are dangerous for babies.
- Avoid taking baby into crowds, like malls and movie theaters, for the first few months.

Hand washing – An easy way to protect baby

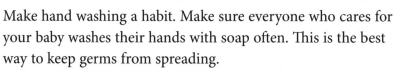

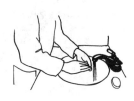

Make hand washing a habit. Make sure everyone who cares for your baby washes their hands with soap often. This is the best way to keep germs from spreading.

- Wash your hands before feeding, touching, or playing with your baby, or mixing formula for a bottle.
- Wash hands after using the bathroom, changing diapers, handling raw foods, blowing your nose, or caring for pets.
- Wash hands more often if you are sick.
- Wash after going to the store or getting gas.
- Make sure older kids wash after coming home from school or playing outside. They should not touch the baby if they are sick.
- Wash your baby's hands before they eat or go to bed. Wash after they play on the floor. Wash if baby puts their hand near their bottom during a diaper change.

How to wash your hands well

1. Use warm water and soap.
2. Rub soapy hands together for 15 to 20 seconds (the time it takes to hum the "Happy Birthday" song slowly). It can take that long to get the germs out of finger nails and creases.
3. Rinse and dry with a clean towel.

Use hand sanitizers, not "anti-bacterial" soaps

If you can't wash with plain soap and water every time, use a hand sanitizer without water. Hand gels and sprays are made with alcohol. They do a good job of killing most germs.

Don't use any cleaners that say they are anti-bacterial. First, they do **not** kill the viruses that cause most sickness. Also, these cleaners can lead to growth of super-germs that antibiotics can't fight. That means if you get sick later on, antibiotics may not help.

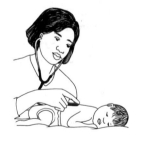

Baby's well-child checkups

Your baby's doctor will want to see baby for their first checkup when they are 3 to 5 days old. After that, well-baby checkups are at 1, 2, 4, 6, 9, and 12 months.

Why does a healthy baby need so many checkups?

Well-baby checkups help keep your baby healthy. The doctor or nurse will check baby's body, growth, and development.

They may spot problems that you can't see. Finding problems early can keep them from getting serious. They will make sure you don't worry more than you need to.

What happens at a well-child checkup?

At each checkup, the provider will weigh your baby and measure their length and head size. They will check ears, eyes, mouth, lungs, heart, belly, penis or vagina, hips, legs, and reflexes.

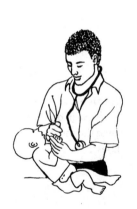

Your baby will get vaccines at most checkups. Different vaccines are given at different ages. (See schedule, page 256.)

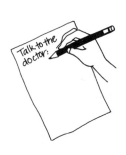

The provider will check your baby's development. They will look for the things baby is learning to do, such as holding up their head and smiling. Be sure to tell baby's provider the new things that you have seen your baby do. You know your baby best. If you worry that baby isn't developing, speak up.

Ask questions

Checkups are the best time to ask the doctor or nurse any questions you have. Bring a list of things you want to talk about to the checkup. Write down what the provider tells you, so you can remember later.

Use the notes page at the end of this chapter to keep track of your baby's early checkups and first vaccines.

Baby's vaccine records

Your clinic or health department will give you a card to keep a record of your baby's checkups and vaccines. You will need this information if you change doctors. When your child goes to child care or school, you will need to know the vaccines they have had. Keep the card in a safe place. Bring it to all your baby's checkups.

Ask your provider if they use an **IIS (Immunization Information System)**. An IIS keeps all of your vaccine records in one place.

Vaccines fight deadly diseases

Why do babies need vaccines?

Your baby needs vaccines to protect them from some very serious diseases like measles, diphtheria, polio, and tetanus. These germs spread very easily and can be very serious. Before vaccines, many people died from these illnesses. Many more people were left with lifelong disabilities like deafness or trouble walking.

When your baby gets a vaccine, their body makes cells to fight those germs. These cells make baby immune to (very unlikely to catch) those diseases. Thanks to vaccines, few people get these diseases today. Because of this, many people don't know how serious they can be.

*Outbreak: When a lot of people in one area catch the same illness.

But outbreaks* still happen. There have been more and more outbreaks of measles and pertussis (whooping cough). This happens because people who *do not* get the vaccines can catch these germs. Then they carry the germs wherever they go.

Outbreaks of measles really happen

In 2014, there was a big outbreak of measles in the US. Another outbreak in January 2015 started at a crowded theme park. Children who got sick had not had the measles (MMR) vaccine. Schoolmates who also had not had that vaccine had to stay home from school for 21 days.

Measles isn't just a mild sickness with cough and an itchy rash. It can cause many dangerous effects, even death. It can spread four days before a person starts to feel sick. Babies can't get the MMR vaccine until they are a year old, so lots of babies and others are in danger.

Measles isn't the only disease a baby can catch in the US. Babies and others with weak immune systems are safe only when most everyone has had all required vaccines.

These germs spread very easily to others who haven't had the vaccines. This is especially dangerous for:

- Babies too young to get vaccines that are usually given at 6 to 12 months.
- children whose parents decided not to give vaccines to them.
- people with weak immune systems whose bodies can't fight diseases well.

So, giving your baby all vaccines for their age helps protect them and everyone else.

No vaccine for colds

Unfortunately, there is no vaccine for the common cold. So keep babies away from crowds and from people who are coughing, sneezing, or have sore throats.

Get vaccines on time

It's important to get your baby immunized as soon as possible. Don't wait until your child goes to child care or school. There are 12 vaccines made to prevent 16 diseases as of 2024. Some are combined so baby can get fewer shots.

"I was glad to get my baby immunized. Now I don't have to worry that someone might pass a serious illness to my child."

Vaccines and the diseases they prevent

Many of these diseases are rare today. Before vaccines were invented, they were very serious. Most spread through the air by coughing, sneezing, or just breathing. Some are spread by dirty hands or blood from a person who has the germs.

COVID-19 for coronavirus-19, which can cause almost no symptoms or many. It can seem like a mild cold or have severe fever, lung, and body symptoms. It is spread mainly through the air.

DTaP for diphtheria, tetanus, and pertussis.

> **Diphtheria** (dif-thee-ree-a) can cause heart and breathing problems, paralysis, or death. It is spread through the air.

> **Tetanus** (lockjaw) causes severe muscle and breathing problems and, often, death. It spreads through cuts in the skin.

> **Pertussis** (whooping cough) can cause severe coughing, lung problems, seizures, brain damage, or death in babies. It is spread through the air. (An adult or older child with a cough may have pertussis but not feel sick.)

HepA for hepatitis A, a liver disease spreads by stool (poop) in dirty food or water or on hands.

HepB for hepatitis B, another liver disease. It spreads in blood or spit and can pass from mother to baby.

Hib for haemophilus influenzae b (hay-ma-fill-us in-flew-en-zay b), which causes meningitis (brain swelling) and can lead to brain damage or death. It is spread in the air.

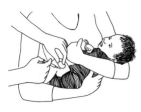

Babies often are given shots in their thighs.

Most vaccines need more than one dose for baby to be fully protected.

Older kids and adults have to get booster shots of some vaccines to stay immune. Some germs change over time. To be able to protect you, the vaccines for these germs change as well.

- ◆ Flu vaccine: this vaccine is different each year to match what types are most common at that time. It is given each year (or "flu season").

- ◆ COVID-19 vaccine: this vaccine is one of the newest. The germs are still changing quickly, so new versions of the

Influenza for "the flu" that comes every fall and winter. It which can be deadly for babies and elders. It spreads through the air.

MMR for measles, mumps, and rubella.

Measles can cause deafness, brain damage, pneumonia (new-mo-nee-ah), or death. It is spread through the air.

Mumps can cause convulsions, deafness, brain damage, or death. It spreads by coughing, sneezing, breathing.

Rubella (German measles) can cause mild sickness in kids. But, if a pregnant woman gets rubella, her baby may be born deaf or blind, or have brain or heart damage. She may also have a miscarriage. Rubella is spread through the air.

PCV for pneumococcal (new-mo-cock-al) disease, which can cause swelling of the brain and spinal cord, blood or lung infections, or death. It spreads through the air.

Polio (IPV) for polio, which can cause life-long paralysis or death. It is spread by stool (poop) on hands or in water.

RSV for respiratory syncytial (sin-SISH-uhl) virus, that peaks in fall and winter. It is spread in the air. RSV is the leading cause of babies needing to be in the hospital. See page 257 to learn more.

RV for rotavirus, which can cause severe vomiting and diarrhea. This leads to loss of a large amount of water, which can cause death. It is spread through stool.

Varicella for chickenpox, which can cause skin rash and brain swelling. Chickenpox can be deadly for babies even if they are not born yet. It is spread through the air or by touching the rash.

vaccine are made often. It is given when new or better vaccines are ready. Some of these are boosters, to keep immunity high.

No vaccine is 100% effective. You may still catch one of these illnesses. But, if you have had your vaccine, your sickness should be shorter and less severe.

You may not like seeing your baby get so many shots. Remember that it only hurts for a little while and it will protect them for many years. To comfort your baby, speak softly, show them a toy, cuddle, or nurse them.

"All six of us got COVID, but the two people who didn't get their boosters got it much worse and it lasted a lot longer."

Outbreaks, epidemics, and pandemics

Some sicknesses, like the flu or a cold, are very common. We expect them to happen to about the same number of people each year. Sicknesses that are not common, we expect not to happen very much or very often. But sometimes, they do.

Outbreak: more cases than expected in a small area.

Epidemic: a very large outbreak in a small area.

Pandemic: a very large outbreak that spreads to a very large area, like COVID-19 did.

An outbreak can happen when people do not get their vaccines. A sickness that stopped happening thanks to a vaccine can come back.

Thanks to vaccines, *measles* had not been a problem in the US since 2000. But, there have been large outbreaks since then. In 2014, someone with the measles went to a crowded theme park. People who were at that theme park took that germ home with them. They spread it everywhere they went. More than half of those cases happened in an area where very few people had gotten vaccines. In 2019, people

Booster shots help keep children's immunity high. Talk with your baby's provider if you have questions about vaccines for your baby.

Special times for vaccines

There are times when your provider may urge you to get more vaccines for your baby. If you travel to a place where certain germs are more common, baby (and you!) may be able to get a vaccine for that. Or, if there is an outbreak of an illness that is risky for baby, they may be able to get an extra dose of a vaccine they've already had.

Stop the spread!

KF94, KN95, and N-95 masks (like those used to slow the spread of COVID-19 during the pandemic) help stop germs from spreading. If you are sick, wearing one of these masks may stop brought the germ with them from other countries where measles still happens. Once in the US, the germ reached people who were at high risk of illness and it spread quickly. This was the worst outbreak in decades.

This can also happen when a germ spreads that there is no vaccine for.

In 2019, **COVID-19** made people very sick in one place. In just a few months, it had spread all over the world. This global pandemic spread faster than doctors or scientists could learn about it. The germ kept making new variants (forms) that spread much more easily and were harder to stop. Hundreds of millions of people around the world got sick. Millions of people died. Many others had symptoms that will last for many years.

The COVID-19 vaccine was created to try to stop the spread. The vaccines and boosters changed to keep up with the changing germs. The more people got the vaccine, the less people got really sick. The global emergency ended in 2023, but the cases of COVID-19 still go up and down quickly. Someday, it may be as predictable as the flu or a cold. But it is still important for everyone to keep up with their vaccines.

Keeping babies in mind. Many vaccines cannot be given to baby in the first month of life. The best thing you can do to protect baby is to **make sure you and others in baby's life get their vaccines**. Stay away from people who could be sick or have been around people who could be. And wash those hands!

you from sharing germs with your baby. Keep a few by your door and ask anyone* who may be sick to either put on a mask or not come in.

*Never put a mask on any child under 2 years old.

Common questions about vaccines

Learning the truth about vaccines can be confusing. A lot of scary things you hear about them on the Internet or in the news are not true. Check the vaccine resources in chapter 17 for the facts about common worries.

Can my baby get vaccines even if they have a cold? It is almost always OK for your baby to get vaccines when they are mildly sick. But, it's good to tell their provider they're sick first.

What if we miss a well-baby checkup? Make another appointment and go in soon so you can keep your baby's immunizations up-to-date.

Vaccines recommended by age 2 as of 2024

Age when usually given	Vaccine name
Birth	HepB, RSV (0–6 months, see below)
2 months	HepB (1–2 months), DTaP, PCV, Hib, Polio, RV
4 months	DTaP, PCV, Hib, Polio, RV
6 months	HepB (6–18 months), DTaP, PCV, Hib, Polio (6–18 months), RV
12–15 months	MMR, PCV, Hib, Varicella, HepA (12-23 months)
15–18 months	DTaP
Other vaccines	**Range of months when it can be given**
COVID-19	Babies should get first dose at 6 months. When they should get the rest of the shots and boosters depends on which brand of vaccine they get.
Influenza (flu)	Babies 6 months and older should get 1–2 doses each fall or winter.
RSV	Babies 6 months and younger should get one dose. When to get it depends on what month baby is born and if/when you got your RSV vaccine while pregnant.
Other vaccines or boosters will be given to school-age children and teens. Special shots may be needed if your baby is bitten by an animal or travels to other parts of the world where other diseases are common.	

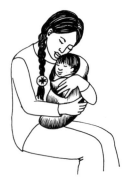

What side effects could my baby have after vaccines? Some will give your baby no side effects. Others may make your baby's arm or leg red or puffy where the shot was given. Baby may get a fever or be fussy for a few days. Ask the doctor or nurse how to comfort your baby and what reactions you should call about.

Is it bad for baby to get so many vaccines at one time? No, but it can be hard for parents to watch. Each shot does hurt for a short time after it's given.

Can a baby get really sick from a vaccine? It is very, very rare for a baby to have a severe reaction. Rumors about problems caused by vaccines have been found to be not true. However, if your baby seems to be sick after getting a vaccine, be sure to call the doctor or nurse.

If I do not want my child to get a vaccine required for child care or school, can they still go? Each state has different laws. In many states, a child who is not immunized can go if parents sign a state waiver form. If an outbreak of disease happens, the child would have to stay home until it's over.

Not being immunized could be dangerous for your child and others. Parents must understand that a child who does not get all their vaccines could catch a serious, preventable illness. They also could spread that illness to others easily.

When baby is sick

If your baby looks or behaves differently than normal

You will soon learn what is normal for your baby. Many babies don't get sick in the first three months. If you are worried, it is best to talk with baby's provider. If your health plan or provider has a phone number for medical advice, you could call it. Providers expect new parents to call as often as they need to.

The only silly questions are the ones you don't ask.

Nights and weekends, if you cannot reach your doctor or nurse, call an urgent care center or after-hours clinic. If it seems serious, take your baby to an emergency room. If you think your baby's life could be in danger, call 9-1-1.

Two baby illnesses to know about

Newborn jaundice

Too much bilirubin in the blood that makes a new baby's skin turn yellow. Most jaundice is mild and goes away soon. If you are breastfeeding, nurse baby as often as possible in the first few days. If it gets worse (or your baby's eyes and hands look yellow) between newborn checkups, call the doctor or nurse. Serious jaundice can lead to brain damage if it is not treated.

RSV

RSV is a that starts like a cold but gets much worse quickly. Baby's lungs could fill with mucus, making it very hard to breathe. Call the doctor right away if baby has a fever, thick green or gray mucus from their nose, heavy breathing, wheezing, or a cough. (It is easy to catch RSV from crowds of people or things a sick person has touched.)

Fever – Taking your baby's temperature

If your baby has a fever, it means their body is fighting off an illness.

Any fever in a baby younger than 2 months old could be serious. If you think your baby has one, call their provider right away. But first, take baby's temperature. You can't know your baby has a fever just by feeling their forehead.

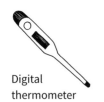

Digital thermometer

There are several kinds of thermometers that you can use for a baby. The most common and cheapest is digital. Others are for use on the forehead or in the ear. Forehead strips and pacifier thermometers do not give a true temperature. (Old-fashioned glass thermometers should not be used.)

There are four ways to take a baby's temperature. They give different readings for a fever. Practice taking your baby's temperature when they are not sick. This will give you an idea of what their normal temperature is. The different ways are:

In the bottom (rectal) with a digital thermometer. It gives the best reading for kids under age 3. 100.4°F (38°C) or higher is a fever and you should call your baby's provider.

How to do it: Put a bit of petroleum jelly on the end of a clean digital thermometer. Lay baby on their back. Bend their knees to their chest with your hand on the back of their thighs to keep them still. Gently put the tip of the thermometer into baby's bottom ½ to 1 inch. Going in too far will hurt them. Gently pull the thermometer out when it beeps.

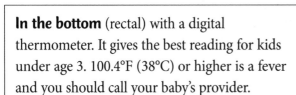

Taking rectal temperature in baby's bottom

In the armpit (axillary) which is not very accurate, but good for a quick check. Use a digital thermometer. With this method, 99°F (37.2°C) is a fever and you should take it again rectally or call baby's provider.

How to do it: Lift your baby's arm and put the tip of the digital thermometer into their armpit. Lower their arm and hold it down against their body until the thermometer beeps.

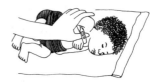

Taking baby's temperature in the armpit

Across the forehead (temporal artery). Using a special thermometer, is good for babies under 3 months old. A fever is 100.4°F (38°C) or higher.

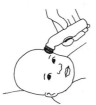

Forehead
(temporal artery)
thermometer

In the ear (tympanic). Using a special thermometer, only for babies older than 6 months. A fever is 100.4°F (38°C) or higher.

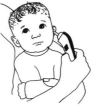

Ear
(tympanic)
thermometer

Ask your health care provider which way they think is best. Ask how high it should be before you call. When you report baby's temperature, be sure to tell which way you took it. The armpit is often the easiest place to take a baby's temperature. It works to get a basic temperature, but rectal is better for an exact reading.

Giving medicine to baby

Most of the time, a baby with a fever will be just fine without medicine. Fevers help their body fight off germs. But, if a fever gets too high (see warning signs) or baby is having a hard time, it may be time for some infant fever medicine (acetaminophen).

Before giving any kind of medicine to your baby, ask a provider or call a nurse hotline. Make sure the medicine is safe for your baby's age and size. Some medicine, like aspirin or cough syrup, should **never** be given to a baby. Other medicines, like ibuprofen, should not be given until baby's at least 6 months old.

Make sure you follow the directions to give the right amount of medicine. This usually depends on the baby's weight and age.

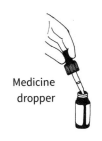

Medicine
dropper

Most baby medicine is a liquid. Use the dropper or medicine syringe (sir-INJ) that comes with it. If you don't have one, you can ask for one at the drug store. Follow the directions to measure carefully. Squirt the medicine in the side of baby's mouth, between their tongue and cheek.

Medicine
syringe

Warning signs—First few months

Any of these signs could mean your baby is very sick. Call right away if your baby has:

- **Yellow skin or eyes** (jaundice), most likely in the first two to three weeks.
- **Infection** of the umbilical cord or circumcised penis: pus* or bright red blood and a red area around the cord stump or tip of the penis.
- **Temperature** under about 97°F (36.1°C) or over 99°F (37.2°C) (when taken in the armpit) or over 100.4°F (38°C) (taken rectally). Always use a thermometer, not your hands, to decide if your baby has a fever.
- **No appetite**: if baby doesn't want the breast or bottle for two feedings in a row.
- **No wet diapers** in 12 hours or less than six wet diapers in 24 hours. (It can be hard to tell if a disposable diaper is wet. Putting a tissue inside it helps you know if it gets wet.)
- **Bloody poops or none at all, or very hard ones.**
- **Vomiting with force** (shooting 2 or 3 feet out of baby's mouth) or for more than 6 hours.
- **Diarrhea** (die-ah-ree-ah): two or more poops that are smelly and watery (and often green), or more than 8 soft stools in 24 hours.
- **Hard tummy** that feels very full.
- **Thick, yellow-green mucus** in baby's nose.
- **Oozing liquid or blood** coming from any opening. (Tiny drops of milk from baby's breasts or blood from the vagina are normal in the first week.)

*Pus: Gooey, smelly, white or yellow discharge from an infected cut.

Some medicine comes as a suppository, which is like a pill that goes into baby's bottom. The medicine melts into baby's body. This is easier than swallowing liquid.

Warning about antibiotics

An antibiotic drug is only useful for certain kinds of illness. If the doctor prescribes one, be sure to give it to baby as long as it says on the bottle. Stopping it too soon may make it work less well the next time your baby needs it.

- ◆ **Breathing problems:**
  - ▪ **Breathing too fast**—more than 60 breaths per minute (babies normally breathe much faster than adults do)
  - ▪ **Very heavy breathing**, having a hard time breathing (baby's skin pulls in around the ribs when they breathe)
  - ▪ **Flared nostrils (open wide), wheezing, grunting**
  - ▪ **No breaths** for more than 15 seconds
  - ▪ **Coughing** that doesn't go away or makes it hard for baby to breathe
- ◆ **Bluish skin**, lips, tongue, or white toes and fingertips (except when baby is cold or crying hard)
- ◆ **More crying** than usual, especially high-pitched shrieks
- ◆ **Sleepier** than usual, little movement, very floppy body
- ◆ **Jittery** or shaky movements
- ◆ **Hearing problem** if baby does not notice loud noises

It's always better to call than to just worry.

Before calling the doctor

- ◆ Take your baby's temperature if you think they have a fever. Write down how high it is, how you took it, and at what time.
- ◆ Write down what is making you worry (for example: pale skin, screaming cry, no stools, vomiting, or diarrhea).
- ◆ Have a pencil and paper ready when you call. Use these to write down what the doctor or nurse tells you.

Call your provider's office or a consulting nurse. They will tell you what you can do at home to help your baby feel better. They may ask you to bring your baby into the office or go to an urgent-care clinic or emergency room.

Use antibiotics only for what the doctor prescribes them for. They do not help colds or the flu. Using an antibiotic when it is **not** needed is not good for baby or for you.

Keep track of your baby's checkups and immunizations on the last page of the chapter.

Follow directions for storing medicines. Some need to be kept in the refrigerator. Store all drugs out of reach of children.

Taking care of baby teeth

It is important to keep baby teeth healthy. Your baby needs those teeth for many things besides chewing food. Teeth help baby talk. They also hold space in the gums for their second set of teeth.

As soon as their first teeth come in, use a soft baby toothbrush with a tiny smear (like a grain of rice) of kid's fluoride toothpaste.

Tips for partners

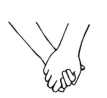

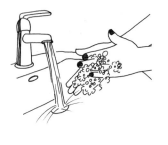

- Help make sure your baby gets to all of their checkups. Go to checkups when you can. It is the best way for you to know what baby's provider says.

- Make sure your own vaccines are up to date. Take care of yourself so you don't get sick. Young babies often get germs from their parents or other caregivers.

- Wash your hands often. Use soap. Scrub front and back, between fingers, and under nails.

- If you have been around a sick person or anything dirty, change your clothes before you hold baby.

- Limit guests. Don't invite anyone who may be sick to visit while baby is new.

- Learn the warning signs (earlier in this chapter) so you know how to tell when your baby is sick.

- Make sure the 24-hour phone number for their doctor or nurse is in your phone.

- Know where the nearest urgent-care clinic or emergency room is.

Your baby's first checkups

Newborn screening

____ Hearing screen

____ First blood screen (before going home)

____ Second blood screen (if required in your state) in the second week

____ Heart screen (CCHS)

____ Bilirubin screen

Comments: _____

_____

Remember: follow up on any screens that show the need for other tests.

Well-baby checkups

(The exact schedule will depend on your baby's health and on your health care provider or insurance plan.)

Questions you may want to ask at the next checkup:

How does my baby's height and weight compare with that of other babies? or *What percentile is my baby in?*

_____

_____

_____

First checkup (three to five days) (date) _____

Baby's age ____ weeks; weight ____ pounds, ____ ounces;

Length ____ inches; head size ____ inches

Comments: _____

Date and time of next checkup: _____

Questions you may want to ask at the next checkup:

Does my baby need extra Vitamin D?

How is my baby developing?

_____

_____

_____

Second checkup (1 month) (date) _____

Baby's age _____ weeks; weight _____ pounds, _____ ounces;

Length _____ inches; head size _____ inches

Comments: _____

_____

Third checkup (2 months) (date) _____

Baby's age _____ weeks; weight _____ pounds, _____ ounces;

Length _____ inches; head size _____ inches

Comments: _____

_____

Date and time of next checkup
(usually at 4 months): _____

First vaccines baby has been given

First doses of vaccines	Dates given
Hep B: first at birth	_____
DTaP: first at 2 months	_____
Polio: first at 2 months	_____
Hib: first at 2 months	_____
PCV: first at 2 months	_____
RSV: first at birth or just before RSV season	_____
RV: first at 2 months	_____

Keep a permanent, long-term record of vaccines or immunizations on a form from your doctor or nurse or clinic. You will need it to show your child care and school district the shots that baby has had.

Chapter 16

Taking Care of Yourself

Remember to take care of your own health! Your body and mind need to recover from giving birth so you can take good care of your baby.

For the first few weeks after birth, you need plenty of rest and time to get to know your baby. It's okay if all you want to do now is eat, sleep, and care for your baby. Those are your most important jobs right now. Of course, if you have other young kids, also spend at least a little time with them.

Let your family and friends help out now. You may need to tell them what would be most helpful. Sometimes a person

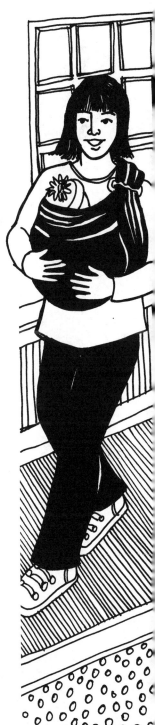

wants to help but makes you feel stressed out. Ask them to do things out of the house. Ideas would be walking the dog, doing food shopping, or cooking food to bring over.

Keeping the stress down at home

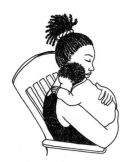

Don't worry too much about house work. Just let the dust pile up for a while. Let other people help with things like laundry, making dinner, doing the dishes, and cleaning the bathroom. They could hold baby while you take a shower and eat.

It's nice to have loved ones come to visit, but let them know to keep it short. You should feel OK about saying that it's time for you and baby to take a nap. Don't feel like you need to entertain people or take care of others right now. It is also okay to say "no visitors today" or ask people to leave meals or gifts outside the door.

A home visit from a nurse

Some health programs or clinics may offer a visit from a nurse a few days after you get home. Ask your provider about this. If you can get it, it is a wonderful service. A nurse would come to see how you both are doing. They would answer questions about your baby's needs and your recovery. They could give you hands-on help with baby care and breastfeeding. See page 294 for a list of programs.

What to expect as your body heals

- ◆ **Birth can make you very tired.** You may ache or feel sore. Talk to your provider about pain medicine that is safe for you now. Taking it on time will help you rest and heal.

- ◆ **You will have discharge** from your vagina for a few weeks. Use pads only, not tampons. At first, it will be heavy and bright red, and may have clots (thick blobs). Then, it should slow down and turn pink or brown.

- ◆ **If the discharge** turns bright red again, you should rest more. If the bleeding gets heavier, see warning signs on the next page, then call your provider right away.

- **Your uterus will start to shrink.** Use the Kegel squeeze and the pelvic tilt (page 28) to help your vagina and tummy get back in shape.

- **You may have cramps,** especially when you are nursing. If they get very painful or make you feel sick, call your provider.

- **If you had an episiotomy or tear,** you will be sore. Keep the area clean. Change your pad often. Soak in a very shallow (sitz) bath or use witch hazel pads (from the drug store) or cold packs. Make cold packs by soaking maxi pads in water or witch hazel and cooling them in the freezer.

- **Eating foods with fiber helps to prevent constipation.** There is lots of fiber in fresh fruits and vegetables, bran cereal, and dried apricots or prunes. Also, drink at least 8 to 12 glasses of water a day. Your provider may also advise using stool softener pills.

"I tried eating lots of fruits and veggies but I was still constipated. When I started drinking lots of water, too, it worked better. Prune juice worked really well."

- **If you had a tear or stitches from an episiotomy,** sitting down or going to the bathroom may be painful. Hard chairs may be easier for sitting. When sitting down on the toilet, squeeze your cheeks (buttocks) together, then sit. Spread your legs to both sides of the toilet for more comfort.

- **If it's hard to pee (urinate),** drink lots of water. Try to pee when you are in the shower. While sitting on the toilet, squirt warm water on the area. If pee doesn't come out, call your doctor or midwife.

- **While pooping (pushing stool out),** hold some toilet paper or a witch hazel pad against the stitches and press up to protect the stitches. Wipe from front to back and clean your bottom carefully.

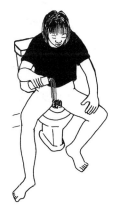

Squirt warm water around your vagina to make peeing easier.

- **Put nothing into your vagina for at least six weeks.** That means no sex or tampons. Don't forget to get—and use—contraceptives (birth control) when you start having sex.

Healing after a cesarean birth

If you have a c-section, most of the things listed above will apply to you. But there are a few more things to know.

- **You will hurt for a while.** It takes four to six weeks for the cut to heal. You will have a checkup six weeks afterward.

- **Take care of your incision (cut).** Ask the doctor or nurse how to keep it clean and when you can get it wet. Be gentle with it, no scrubbing or clothes that rub against it. Watch for signs of infection—if it feels hot, turns bright red, oozes, or opens up, you need to call your doctor.

- **Get lots of rest.** It takes longer to heal if you get overtired. Rest as much as you can. Use your energy to feed and cuddle your baby.

- **Don't lift** anything heavier than your baby for the first few weeks. Keep the things you need within easy reach.

- **Find ways of holding baby** that don't press on the cut. Put a pillow on your belly when holding baby in your lap. Or try the football hold—baby's body goes under your arm and their feet are behind you.

- **Get some gentle exercise every day.** Deep breathing, stretching, and walking are enough at first. Talk to your doctor or midwife about what is safe.

- **To lessen pain when you sit up**, stand up, sit down, or bend over, press a firm pillow over your stitches. Press your hand (or the pillow) over the incision when you laugh, cough, sneeze, or move suddenly. It will help limit the pain.

- **Ask your doctor or midwife** when it is safe to use stairs, exercise more, or drive. Accept all offers to help around the house with cooking, cleaning, and the laundry.

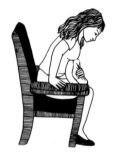

Hold a pillow over your stitches when you get up. This will make it less painful to get up.

Warning Signs – The First Few Weeks

Call your provider if you have:

- Heavy bleeding—blood clots bigger than an egg or bright red blood that soaks your menstrual pad in an hour or less.
- Discharge from your vagina that smells bad.
- Fever of 100.4°F (38°C) or higher or flu-like symptoms.
- Trouble urinating or having bowel movements.
- Pain near or in your vagina, bottom, or belly.
- Signs of infection (pus, redness, soreness, or swelling) from your stitches (from a c-section, episiotomy, or tear).
- Pain in your breasts; breast that have warm areas; nipples that are cracked or very sore.
- Swelling in one or both legs, or a warm, painful area in one leg.
- Feeling very emotional or sad. Having trouble sleeping. See the section of moods later in this chapter.

Breast care

Your breasts will keep changing after you have your baby. Wear a bra or top with good support when you feel like you need it. Other times, you may be more comfortable in something soft or loose. Wear what feels good, especially if your breasts are sore. See chapter 12 for tips on breast care while breastfeeding, formula feeding, or both.

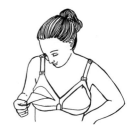

A bra with good support

Keep up your healthy habits

Follow the healthy food habits you started in pregnancy (chapter 4). You need to eat well to get back your strength and energy. Eat plenty of protein and calcium from meat, fish, beans, tofu, nuts, seeds, milk, and cheese. If you are breastfeeding twins or triplets, you will need to eat more to make larger amounts of breast milk.

Start exercising gently

Protect your back. Keep a straight back and bend your knees when lifting your baby. Try to stand up straight when you carry them. Make sure the baby carrier you use has good back support for you and fits baby well, too. Other exercises will help, too, like those shown in the pictures.

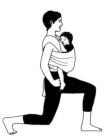

You could take baby with you to an exercise class for new moms.

Walking is the best way to start getting back in shape. You can wear your baby in a carrier. They'll like the ride and the gentle movement. If you had a c-section, ask your doctor before starting any exercise.

Continue to avoid alcohol and other drugs

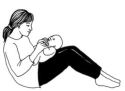

Sit with baby on your thighs, then lean back slowly with a straight back.

Being a parent can be hard, but using alcohol, cigarettes, and other drugs doesn't make it easier. They can make it harder for you to handle the tough parts of parenting.

If you are breastfeeding, these drugs can hurt your baby's brain and growth. Breast milk carries alcohol, nicotine, and other drugs to your baby.

Smoke in the air can give baby problems, too. Babies of smokers have more colds, ear infections, and a higher risk of SIDS. Anyone who smokes should do so outside the house and not in the car with baby.

E-cigarettes may not be much healthier than regular cigarettes. Little is known about the vapor that goes into the air. The liquid inside or in refills is very poisonous to kids who might touch it or drink it.

Your own checkups after birth

Baby's first checkups are very important, but so are your own! Your provider will want to talk to you by phone or in person in the first few days after baby is born.

Your provider will want to check in with you:

- ◆ 1 to 3 days after birth, by phone or in person.
- ◆ 1 to 2 weeks after birth, if any special care is needed.
- ◆ 6 weeks after birth, in person, for a full checkup.
- ◆ Up to 12 weeks, if more care or support is needed.

After that, get your checkup each year to make sure your body adjusts well.

In these first few months after giving birth, your provider will want to know how you are doing. They will ask about these things:

- **Self care:** Are you eating and sleeping?
- **Habits:** Do you need help with not smoking? Are you being active?
- **Bleeding:** Are you bleeding less? Do you have worries about smell or color?
- **Healing:** How is your tear or incision? Do you have pain?
- **Bladder and bowels:** Any problems peeing or pooping?
- **Emotions:** How are you feeling? Do you have support?
- **Breastfeeding:** How is nursing going? How much is baby eating? What questions do you have?
- **Breast care:** Do you have pain, redness, or bleeding? Do you need help making more or less milk?
- **Sex life:** Do you want to have sex? Are you worried about sex? What is your plan for birth control?
- **Safety:** Are you and baby in a safe place? Do you have what you need? Do you need support?

These visits are a great time to ask questions. No worry is too small and having answers can help you feel less stressed. Your provider can also help connect you with all kinds of resources and support.

Sex after baby is born

Wait until you're ready

Everyone is different when it comes to having sex after baby's birth. Some people are ready for sex after just a few weeks. Others don't feel ready for a few months or more. It is a good idea to wait at least six weeks before having sex or putting anything in your vagina. This gives your body time to heal inside. It also gives you time to take care of the rest of your body and all its changes.

Abstinence – Having no sex

Abstinence can mean different things to different people. For some, it means not having any kind of sex with another person. This also prevents STIs. For other people, it means not having penis-vagina sex. In these first weeks, abstinence gives your body time to heal. It also keeps you from getting pregnant.

There are many reasons people don't feel ready for sex, even after six weeks

- Your body and feelings are very tired from taking care of your baby.
- Sex can seem scary when your body (vagina, bottom, or c-section cut) is sore or healing.
- Your breasts may be leaky or sore. Or just tired of being touched.

It's okay to need more time. Masturbation may be one way to get to know your own body again. And there are other ways to be close with your partner, like cuddling, massage, or kissing. Using your hands or mouth on your partner's body (or theirs on yours) can be a gentle way to enjoy sexual feelings.

Talk to your partner and take things slow. If you still don't feel ready for sex after a few months, tell your provider. It could be a sign of other problems, like vaginal discomfort or postpartum depression.

Family planning

There are so many things to think about when planning for your family. Now is the time to start thinking ahead. How many kids do you want to have? When do you want to have them? Think about what support you have and how you would move forward with your schooling or career. Do you have a partner who you plan to be with for a long time? Talk to them about their goals for your family and the future. It's important to think about the hard stuff as well as the fun stuff.

"My friend had two kids under 2 years old at the same time. Her oldest had such a hard time. I don't want to get pregnant again that soon!"

It is usually best to wait at least 18 months to get pregnant again. This gives your body time to heal and makes it more likely that your next baby will be healthy. In the meantime, it's important to come up with a plan to prevent pregnancy. This is called birth control.

Plan ahead for birth control

The best time to decide on birth control is *before* you start having penis-vagina sex again. There are many types of birth control. Some must be used every time you have sex. Others must be taken on a schedule, even if you don't have sex. Some can last weeks, months, or even years.

If you or your partner are having sex with more than one person, you may also need to think about sexually transmitted infections (STIs). Condoms are the only type of birth control that protect against any STIs.

To decide what birth control method may be best for you, think about:

Some types of birth control can be started right after birth. Then you don't have to worry about getting pregnant when you do feel ready to have sex again.

- ◆ How well does it prevent pregnancy?
- ◆ How easy is it to use?
- ◆ How soon can you use it?
- ◆ How easy is it to get?
- ◆ Does it also prevent sexually transmitted infections (STIs)?
- ◆ Can you use it while breastfeeding?
- ◆ Is there any other reason it might not be a good fit for you?

Birth control options

Hormonal birth control – Must use on a schedule

Some methods of birth control use hormones to prevent pregnancy. These hormones tell your body not to ovulate. They may also thicken the mucus on your cervix to make it harder for the sperm to get through. The hormone IUD and shot both last a long time with no effort on your part. Other hormone methods (see next page) must be taken on a strict schedule or they will not work. But, when used properly, they prevent pregnancy over 90 percent of the time. These **do not** protect against any STIs.

Oral contraceptives (the pill)

A hormone pill that prevents ovulation. Must be taken at the same time every day to prevent pregnancy. Some medicines and herbs can make your pill not work. Be sure to ask your provider about any other medicines you take. Use a backup method, like a condom or a sponge, when needed.

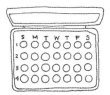

LARC—Long-acting reversible contraception

If you know you don't want to get pregnant anytime soon, LARC may be a good choice for you. LARC options include an implant, IUD, or injection. These are the most effective birth control and prevent pregnancy almost 100% of the time. They are also the easiest to use. They do require a prescription and a visit to your provider to have it put in. But, once it's in, you will not get pregnant for months, or even years, until it runs out or is removed. This **does not** protect against any STIs.

Implant: a small (match-stick sized) rod placed under the skin on your arm. It releases hormones to prevent pregnancy for up to 5 years. When you want to get pregnant, a provider must remove it.

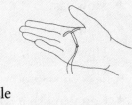

IUD (intrauterine device): a small device that sits in your uterus to block sperm from getting to the egg. Some release hormones to prevent pregnancy (see below). Another IUD uses copper to keep sperm away. An IUD must be put in by your provider, then lasts for 3 to 12 years without much hassle for you. When you want to get pregnant, a provider can remove it.

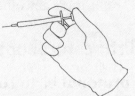

Injection: a shot of hormone that prevents pregnancy for up to 3 months. It works very well, as long as you get them on time.

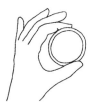

Vaginal ring

A small, flexible ring that sits inside your vagina. Some are replaced with a new one each month, and you choose if you want a period in between. Others are taken out, washed, and put back in a week later, after your period.

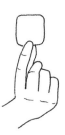

Patch

A small patch you stick to your skin. Each patch lasts one week if applied correctly. Make sure you follow all rules about where to apply and when you change.

Barriers – Must use every time.

Barrier methods prevent pregnancy by keeping sperm away from your cervix. These work well if you always use it correctly, each time you have sex. Some, like a diaphragm or cervical cap, must be fitted by a provider. But others, like condoms, can be bought at the store. All of them can be put in and taken out on your own at home.

External condoms – Protect against some STIs

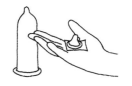

A stretchy tube that covers the penis. Prevents pregnancy by catching the semen (cum) so it can't enter the vagina. A new condom must be put on an erect (hard) penis before sex each time. It must be removed carefully after sex so it does not tear or spill.

Internal condoms – Protect against some STIs

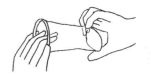

A loose, stretchy tube that is placed inside the vagina (or anus). It has a ring to help put it in and to hold it in place. Like other condoms, it prevents pregnancy by keeping the semen out of the vagina and protects against many STIs. It also must be placed before sex and handled carefully in order to work properly.

Diaphragm or cervical cap

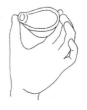

A soft cover that fits over your cervix. When used with spermicide, it prevents pregnancy by blocking the cervix and slowing the sperm down. It must be put in place before you have sex and can stay in for 24 hours. If you have sex more than once in that time, add more spermicide in your vagina before each time. Be sure to follow the instructions on how long to leave it in after sex and when to take it out. Once removed, it can be washed and used again. These methods must be just the right size and shape to work properly. If you have one from before you were pregnant, it may no longer fit your cervix well. It's important to have it fitted by a provider.

Sponge

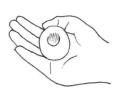

A small plastic sponge that covers your cervix. It has spermicide* in it that you release by getting it wet. Once foamy, you put the sponge deep into your vagina, and it will work for 24 hours. Be

---

***Spermicide:** a thick cream, gel, film, or foam that you put deep inside your vagina before sex. It helps prevent pregnancy by blocking the cervix and using a chemical to slow down the sperm. Used by itself, it prevents pregnancy almost 80 percent of the time. But, using it with another method, like a condom, adds protection.

sure to follow the rules for how long to leave it in after sex and when to take it out. It cannot be reused.

Breastfeeding as birth control?

Breastfeeding in the first six months can prevent pregnancy in some people. Nursing may stop your body from ovulating (releasing an egg), but only if:

- ◆ you nurse baby every 4–5 hours, day and night.
- ◆ baby is only eating your breastmilk, no formula or food.
- ◆ your period has not come back yet since giving birth.

If any of these things are not true, your body may release an egg. If you really do not want to get pregnant, it is important to use a more effective type of birth control.

Permanent birth control – Sterilization

If you know you will not ever want more babies, ask your provider about sterilization. These surgeries are fairly easy and are more than 99 percent effective at preventing pregnancy. Once your provider says you are healed and ready after the sterilization, you will not get pregnant. **This does NOT protect against STIs.**

Tubal ligation (having your tubes tied)

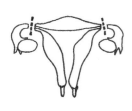

A surgery that blocks or removes the tubes that carry your eggs to your uterus. This prevents pregnancy because your eggs will never come down to where sperm could reach them. You may be able to have this done right after birth, so all of your healing happens at once.

Vasectomy

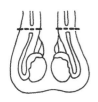

A simple surgery that blocks or cuts the tubes that carry sperm to the penis. After a few months, a doctor will check to make sure there is no sperm in the semen (cum). Once the semen is sperm-free, there is almost no risk of pregnancy.

Emergency Contraception

It is best to use birth control before you have sex. But, if that doesn't work, you need birth control that works after you have sex. This is called **emergency contraception (EC)**.

IUD

Having an approved IUD put in within five days of unprotected sex is the most reliable form of EC. They put it in and that's it. You won't get pregnant for up to 12 years unless you have it removed. It can be hard to get an appointment soon enough, so be sure to call right away.

Morning-after pill

Taking an EC pill (ECP) within five days of unprotected sex is the easiest form of EC. You can get ECPs from most drug stores without a prescription, so you don't have to wait. ECPs work by delaying ovulation. The sooner you take it, the better it works. But, if an egg has already been released, ECPs cannot stop pregnancy from happening. They also don't work well for people over 165–195 lbs.

Unprotected sex – What if . . .?

What if we pull the penis out before it ejaculates (cums)?

Any fluid from the penis can have sperm in it before, during, or after an orgasm*. Pulling out (the withdrawal method) may make pregnancy less likely, but it does not prevent it.

*Orgasm:** The peak of good sexual feelings and sudden release of sexual tension. Often leads to ejaculation (cumming).

What if I go pee right after sex?

During sex, semen goes into your vagina. Pee comes out of a different hole, called the urethra. So, peeing after sex is healthy and can help prevent infection, but does not prevent pregnancy.

What if I shower right after sex? Or douche*?

Washing or rinsing will not prevent pregnancy. Once you have semen in your vagina, the sperm quickly move up through your cervix and into your uterus. Rinsing the inside of your vagina (douching) can actually push sperm deeper in. It can also lead to infection and other problems.

*Douche:** To wash out the *inside* of the vagina by squirting liquid into it. Douching is not recommended.

What if I forgot my pill, a condom breaks, or I was forced to have sex without birth control?

Take your missed pill as soon as you can. Look into emergency contraception right away (see above).

If your partner wants you to have unprotected sex, talk to your provider about a birth control method that you are in control of. Some cannot be noticed by partners.

How are you feeling?

Having a new baby changes your life in many ways. It is a very emotional time with highs and lows. For some people it is a happy time but for others it can be very hard. There are so many new things to learn and your baby needs you all the time. It is okay to have mixed feelings.

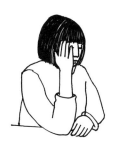

Get help if you start to feel depressed.

Many parents feel upset or sad after their child is born. They may cry easily, get mad over little things, or have trouble eating and sleeping in the first few weeks. This is called the "baby blues" and 8 out of 10 parents go through it. But, if these feelings last longer, get worse, or make it hard for you to care for yourself or your baby, it may be something more serious.

*Mood disorder:
Emotional illness or condition.

*Postpartum:
The time after a baby's birth.

Mood disorders* in pregnancy or after giving birth

Mood disorders happen to many parents during pregnancy or after baby is born. Postpartum* depression and anxiety are the most common, but there are others, too. For some people, this is the first time they have had these problems.

Watch each other for any of the warning signs on page 279. Get help as soon as you feel your mood changing. Try not to hide from it or be a superhero. It's important not to wait.

"After my first baby was born, I spent a whole year being really worried that I wasn't doing everything right. It was awful. With my second baby, I got some medicine for my anxiety. What a difference! I feel like I'm a much better mom now."

It can be hard to admit to or talk about these feelings. It can even be hard to believe that you have a problem. Many people try to just "live with it" or pretend they are okay. Some people need others to get help for them because they are too upset to call for themselves. Remember, this can happen to either parent and is hard on the whole family.

How does a mood disorder happen?

It can happen from too much stress, too little sleep, bad eating habits, money trouble, or family problems. It is more likely if you have had a birth that was very hard, scary, or not what you

Warning Signs – Is It More Than Just Baby Blues?

Please check the things you or your partner feels often, even if they don't feel serious to you. Some may be hard to admit. Be honest with yourself.

Have you had a mood disorder (like depression or anxiety) before?

- ☐ Do you feel very sad?
- ☐ Do you feel mad at the people around you over little things?
- ☐ Is it hard for you to feel close to your baby?
- ☐ Do you feel panic or are you always worried about how you are caring for baby?
- ☐ Is it hard for you to eat or sleep?
- ☐ Do you feel very happy one minute and very upset the next?
- ☐ Do you have bad thoughts in your mind that you can't get rid of?
- ☐ Do you feel like you're "going crazy"?
- ☐ Do you feel like you can't be a good parent?
- ☐ Are you afraid you might hurt yourself or your baby?

If the answer is yes to any one of these, tell your provider. You may have a mood disorder. It can happen to anyone, including dads or partners, and is very common. There is help! You don't need to suffer.

wanted. However, a mood disorder is more common if you or a relative has had depression, anxiety, bipolar, or obsessive-compulsive disorder in the past. It is also more likely if you have been abused, even as a child.

What to do if you're having a hard time

Tell your provider if either you or your partner has any of the signs above. Tell them you want to talk to someone who works with mood disorders. The sooner you get professional help, the better for you and your baby. There is no need to suffer.

Call **1-800-944-4773** to get support from Postpartum International. If you are in crisis and need help right away, call the National Suicide Prevention Hotline at **1-800-273-8255**. In an emergency, call 9-1-1.

If your partner seems depressed

What to say to your partner that can help:

* *You're not alone. I'm here for you.*
* *You will get better. We'll get through this.*
* *This isn't your fault.*
* *I love you so much. The baby loves you so much.*
* *I'm sorry you're hurting.*
* *You're a great parent. I love how you stroke baby's head while nursing.*
* *As your partner gets better, tell them the ways you see them getting better.*

Things people say that are *not* helpful:

* *Snap out of it.*
* *Try feeling happy.*
* *Just calm down.*
* *Think about all you have to be thankful for.*

Ways to help yourself

Take care of yourself

Try to eat well and get some sleep each day (at least four or five hours of nonstop sleep in a row). Get up, move around, and get out of the house. Fresh air and exercise can help with stress.

Remember – this is not your fault

You didn't make this happen. You're not alone. It will get better.

Be around people you like

Just because you love someone doesn't mean he or she is good at helping you feel relaxed. Ask people to visit who make you laugh, whom you trust, and who will support you. Share your feelings, good or bad, with them. Put off stressful visits until you or your partner feels better.

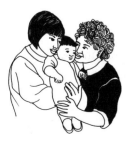

Have a plan for support

Say "yes" when people offer to help. Think of things people can do for you and ask them. It could be something big like helping to pay your bills or something small like bringing a meal or walking your dog.

Talk to others

It helps to know you're not alone. Ask around in your group of friends. Also find a support group in your area or online.

No one is a perfect parent!

Are you or your partner worried about doing things wrong? You do not have to know all the answers. You will learn as you go along. You do not have to do it alone.

You can get advice from friends, relatives, neighbors, your health clinic, and many organizations. There are parent groups, lactation consultants, and playgroups to turn to. There is a lot of information that you can trust in books, videos, and internet sites.

Just remember, you are the parents and get to decide which advice is best for your family.

Tips for partners

This is a big time for you. You are playing a huge role in making sure your partner and baby are taken care of. You also need to make sure that you take care of yourself! Both of you will need to have patience and get rest when you can. There are two big things to pay attention to: sex and depression.

Talking about sex

It can be hard to talk about sex after baby. Go to page 271 and read about sex after baby. Try to think about how much your partner's body has been through. It may seem amazing to you, but it may be exhausting for them. They may feel bad saying that they are too tired or "touched out." They may still be healing and be scared it might hurt.

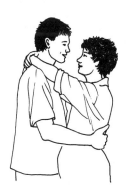

It is okay to show your partner you care and say that you want to be close again. But be patient, don't push. Try other ways of being close for a while.

When you do have sex, be sure to use protection. It's important not to get pregnant again too soon.

More tips for partners

- Read this chapter to learn what your partner is going through after birth. It will help you understand and know how to help.

- Put phone numbers for your partner's provider, baby's doctor, and a lactation consultant in your phone or on the door of the fridge. Offer to call if either of you is worried.

- Find a local group of dads with babies for play or support.

Affirmations for parents to remember

I am learning more every day about being good to myself.

I have friends I can call on when I need support or someone to talk with.

I am being the best parent I can be, knowing what I know now.

Nobody is perfect. My child will forgive any small mistakes I make.

I enjoy seeing how my baby learns and grows from week to week.

I'm not the first person who has been depressed during this time. I can ask for help.

My baby gives me the chance to become a new person.

I am a good parent.

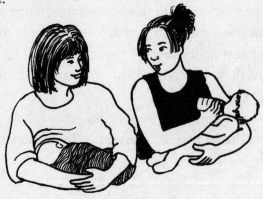

Chapter 17

Resources to Help You

Your health care provider is the best place to ask questions. You can also learn a lot on your own. This book is a great place to learn the basics about pregnancy, birth, postpartum, and baby care. But there's a lot more that may help you to know. This chapter has many links to other places to find information you can trust.

Always talk to your provider about anything new or different you learn. Never make any big changes before asking your provider if it's a good option for you.

Get help right now

If you need help right now, there is help.

You can search online for "(Your state) crisis hotline" to find support in your area. If that does not help, or if you can't search for help, call one of these emergency hotlines from anywhere in the US:

9-1-1 (Emergency services) English and Español

Emergency – when a life may be in danger or there has been a crime. They can send emergency medical, fire, or police services. They can also talk you through what to do while you wait. Available in English and Español. You can text 911 in some places, but not others, and voice calls are always the fastest way to get help.

9-8-8 (Suicide and crisis lifeline) English and Español

Call or text for help with suicide and mental health struggles. All counselors are trained in crisis support. You can also use the menu to choose someone specially trained to help Spanish-speakers, veterans, or LGBTQI+ youth and young adults. After you make your choices, you will be connected to your local crisis center or the one that best meets your needs. 988 Lifeline also uses interpreters to offer help in more than 240 languages.

Find help near you

There are many ways to learn more and find support. Ask your provider about resources in your area or to help you get connected to your local public health clinic.

2-1-1 (through United Way)

Call 2-1-1 to find community resources that help with bills and rent, caregiver support, legal trouble, mental health, and other basic needs. Visit www.211.org to find your local 211 program.

Department of Health

Visit your state's Department of Health website to find what resources they offer. There may be programs for dental care, health care, help with bills, child care, finishing school, drug and alcohol use, safe housing, and other basic needs. Search online for "(Your state) Department of Health."

Public Health Clinic

Call your county's public health clinic and ask about resources. They may have a home visiting program, parent support program, or even a place to get free baby items. Sign up for WIC or financial assistance programs. Get help signing up for insurance or getting prenatal care.

WIC

The WIC program helps low-income pregnant, postpartum, and breastfeeding women, and children up to age 5. WIC provides EBT cards (or vouchers) that can be used to buy food each month to help make sure they get the nutrients they need. It also provides breastfeeding support, and formula for babies who aren't fully breastfed. Most clinics also offer health and vaccine screenings. Learn more or find your local program at www.fns.usda.gov/wic.

Planned Parenthood

Planned parenthood offers many health services, like pelvic exams and cancer screenings. They are experts in sexual health care and provide STD tests, pregnancy tests, and birth control. They provide abortions and support for those who have been through trauma or sexual assault. They are committed to providing affirming care to people of all gender identities and sexual orientations. Free to low-cost care to those who need it, and help signing up for insurance.

Call 1-800-230-7526 or chat online at www.plannedparenthood.org (English and Español).

Text "PPNOW" to 774636 (English) or texto "AHORA" al 774636 (Español).

Visit www.plannedparenthood.org to chat online, find a clinic near you, find an abortion provider, or to learn about many health and safety topics.

> **Beware of Crisis Pregnancy Centers**
> Many programs called "crisis pregnancy center" or "pregnancy aid" are unsafe places to get help.
> See page 6 to learn more.

Other places in your area

Many places in your community may have support programs or keep a list of resources in your area. Some ideas of places to call or visit:

Library	Community college	Hospital
School health center	Health center	Worship or faith center
Community center	Mental health center	

Get more help

You probably use the internet to find all kinds of information and advice. When it comes to health and safety, it is very important to look for information you can trust. Major health and safety agencies (many end in .gov) are sources you can count on. They are kept up to date and are based on science and best practices.

We have gathered a list of helpful resources that you can trust. Many of the sites listed have their own lists of recommended resources, too. If anything looks old, or a link doesn't work, search for that program's name and the topic you're looking for (such as "AAP safe sleep").

When in doubt, talk to your provider about anything you read or hear.

General health and safety

womenshealth.gov

familydoctor.gov

medlineplus.gov

healthychildren.org

kidshealth.org

Help by topic – In order from before pregnancy to after birth
Pregnancy tests and birth control

Planned Parenthood (see page 284)

All needs around sex, pregnancy, birth control, Emergency contraception, abortion, or sexual violence.

www.plannedparenthood.org

Call 1-800-230-7526
or text "PPNOW" to 774636

Bedsider

A science-based non-profit that helps people find birth control, Emergency contraception, abortion, and sexual health care that is right for them.

www.bedsider.org (English)
www.bedsider.org/es (Español)

I am not ready to be a parent.
What do I do?

Many people feel unsure they are ready to have a baby. For many people, support and time help them feel more confident in becoming a parent. The more they learn and talk to people, the more prepared they feel to start a family. Even if it is not perfect, they are able to see a life with baby.

Others just aren't ready to raise a baby. Some common reasons are that they:

◆ can't afford to raise a child (or another child).

◆ don't feel ready to be the kind of parent they want for their child.

◆ got pregnant by sexual assault (rape).

◆ have a partner who is violent or abusive and they want to keep their child safe.

◆ don't feel like they can be a single parent.

◆ have an unsafe living situation or unstable housing.

What are the options

Stay pregnant, place baby for adoption

Adoption is the transfer of parental rights from a child's biological parent(s) to adoptive parent(s). It is permanent and means you no longer have any rights to that child.

Why do people consider adoption?

People who are in many of the situations above decide they are not ready for a baby. If they do not want to have an abortion (see next page), they may choose to find someone else to be the baby's parent(s).

Adoption can happen different ways in different states. You can start making plans while you're pregnant, but an adoption is not legal until after the baby is born.

There are also other care options you may want to learn about. Family preservation, temporary care, crisis nurseries, and kinship care are some types of support that don't require you to permanently give up your parental rights.

See the resources on the next pages to learn more about placing a baby for adoption in your state, and to get support while you make your decision.

End the pregnancy (abortion)

Abortion is when a pregnancy is ended. There are two types of abortion: in-clinic abortion and the abortion pill. Both ways are safe when done with the help of an abortion provider.

Why do people consider abortion?

◆ Wanting to focus on being a good parent to the kids they already have.

◆ Not being ready to be a parent yet.

◆ Needing to finish school or keep working or meet other life goals.

◆ Not wanting to have a baby alone or with the person they are with.

For some, staying pregnant is not an option. This may be because:

◆ the pregnancy is dangerous for their health.

◆ how they got pregnant was violent or otherwise traumatic.

◆ the fetus will not survive the pregnancy or will suffer after birth.

The programs below can help you learn more about your options. They offer support by phone, text, chat, or online. No matter what you choose, you don't have to do it alone.

VIDEOS: Global Health Media

Click on "Family Planning" to see all videos. Click on "All Audiences" and choose "Women and partners."

globalhealthmedia.org

Emergency Contraception

(See page 276.)

You can buy some "morning after pills" without a prescription from a drug store or pharmacy. Call your insurance to see if your plan covers over-the-counter Emergency contraception. Common brands are Plan B One Step® or ella®. If you don't see them on the shelf, ask the pharmacist.

Office of Women's Health Helpline

1-800-994-9662 or
www.womenshealth.gov

Planned Parenthood

1-800-230-7526 or
www.plannedparenthood.org

Options – Abortion and adoption

Planned Parenthood

Provides counseling about all options for pregnancy. Can offer resources for prenatal care and parenting support. Also provides abortion care.

1-800-230-7526 or
www.plannedparenthood.org

All-Options

All about making your own choice about pregnancy.

1-888-493-0092 (talkline) or www.all-options.org

Bedsider (See page 285.)

www.bedsider.org/pregnancy_options

Faith Aloud

For those who have spiritual concerns about making decisions about pregnancy. Offers spiritual care before, during, and even long after pregnancy, parenting, abortion, or adoption. A program of All-Options, Faith Aloud provides safe support no matter what choices you consider or make.

1-888-717-5010 (care line) or www.faithaloud.org

Abortion Finder

How to find safe abortion care and support. Can explain abortion laws where you live and help you find safe abortion care. Has a list you can search for health and emotional support before, during, and after an abortion.

www.abortionfinder.org

National Abortion Federation and Hotline

All about making your own choice about pregnancy. Can explain abortion laws where you live and help you find safe abortion care. Can help with Medicaid or insurance coverage and finding funds to cover an abortion.

1-800-772-9100 (Hotline) or prochoice.org (chat online)

National Council for Adoption

Information to help you understand all the types of adoption. Can explain the process of placing your child for adoption and what your rights are where you live. Offers resources, personal stories, and how to find a trustworthy agency or attorney.

adoptioncouncil.org/expectant-parents

National Network of Abortion Funds

All about making your own choice about pregnancy. Can explain abortion laws where you live and help you find safe abortion care. Can help with Medicaid or insurance coverage and finding funds to cover an abortion.

abortionfunds.org/need-an-abortion

Health insurance

Health Insurance Marketplace

All about state health insurance options. Apply online for Medicaid, Children's Health Insurance Program (CHIP), or basic health insurance. You can also log in and make changes to your current plan.

1-800-318-2596 or www.healthcare.gov

www.healthcare.gov/what-if-im-pregnant-or-plan-to-get-pregnant (All the links to help you with health insurance if you are pregnant or trying to get pregnant, or if you recently gave birth.)

Pregnancy and childbirth

CenteringPregnancy

A type of prenatal care that is relaxed and builds connection. A group of 8–10 pregnant people meet with their provider for 1½ to 2 hours, with belly checks done in private. Learn about prenatal health, labor and birth, breastfeeding, and baby care. Many go on to the CenteringParenting program for parenting support in the first two years. Click on "locations" to see who offers CenteringPregnancy near you.

centeringhealthcare.org/what-we-do/centering-pregnancy

Birth classes

Most hospitals and birth centers offer birth classes. Many offer scholarships for those who cannot pay. Ask your provider what classes they recommend. You can also search here:

ICEA (International Childbirth Education Association)

icea.org

Lamaze

www.lamaze.org

Doulas (see page 76.)

Dona International

www.dona.org

DoulaMatch

Learn all about birth and postpartum doulas. Search for doulas based on where you are and what preferences you have.

Keeps active list of Black and Indigenous doulas by state. Also has list of online childbirth classes.

doulamatch.net

Vaccines in pregnancy

(See chapter 3)

CDC

www.cdc.gov/vaccines-pregnancy

Warning signs – Pregnancy and postpartum

HEAR HER – CDC

www.cdc.gov/hearher

Learn about pregnancy and birth

American Academy of Pediatrics (AAP)

www.healthychildren.org/english/ages-stages/prenatal

Centers for Disease Control and Prevention (CDC)

Health, vaccines, and safety in pregnancy
www.cdc.gov/pregnancy

Evidence Based Birth

evidencebasedbirth.com

It Starts with Mom – March of Dimes

www.marchofdimes.org/itstartswithmom

Nemours KidsHealth

kidshealth.org/en/parents/pregnancy-newborn

Office on Women's Health

womenshealth.gov/pregnancy

VIDEOS: Global Health Media

Click on "childbirth" to see all videos. Click on "All Audiences" and choose "Mothers and caregivers."

globalhealthmedia.org

Emotional and mental health

988 Lifeline – Suicide and Crisis Lifeline

24-hour hotline – Call or text

Voice, text, and chat support in English, Español, and ASL. Voice-call support available in more languages with interpreters, call and say the name of your language.

Call or text 9-8-8

Crisis Text Line

Text HOME to 741741or chat or WhatsApp at www.crisistextline.org

National Maternal Mental Health Hotline

24-hour hotline – Call or text (English and Español)

1-833-TLC-MAMA (1-833-852-6262)

National Safe Haven Alliance

Urgent help for those who need to surrender their baby in a safe place after birth.

Call or text 1-888-510-2229

Postpartum Support International HelpLine

1-800-944-4773 (#1 en Español or #2 English)

Text "Help" to 1-800-944-4773 (English) or texto al 1-971-203-7773 (Español)

Postpartum Support International

www.postpartum.net/get-help

Online Support Groups (Click on "online support groups")

A list of online support groups for people who are, were, or are trying to be pregnant. Many groups have a special focus, such as mental health, birth trauma, BIPOC birthing people, infant loss, dad or partner support, multiples pregnancy, substance abuse recovery, and queer or trans parent support.

Baby care – health and safety

Healthychildren.org
Kidshealth.org
Familydoctor.org

Breastfeeding and breast milk

Breastfeeding USA

Learn about breastfeeding, find a breastfeeding counselor, and see a list of helpful videos on many nursing topics.

breastfeedingusa.org

1-612-293-6622 (warmline) leave a message in English or Español and a trained breastfeeding counselor will call you back to offer support over the phone.

Depression and anxiety during and after pregnancy

If you . . .

- Don't feel like yourself
- Are having trouble controlling your feelings
- Feel overwhelmed but can still take care of yourself and baby

You may . . .

be having mood swings or "baby blues" that are common around pregnancy. Take special care of yourself. Let others help support you or take care of baby. If things don't feel better after a couple of weeks, talk to your provider or call 1-833-TLC-MAMA (1-833-852-6262) or one of the resources in this chapter.

If you . . .

- Have strong anxiety or fear that hits with no warning
- Feel foggy or like a robot, just going through the day
- Aren't interested in things you normally like
- Feel scared around your baby or other kids
- Have scary thoughts that won't go away
- Feel guilty or like you are failing as a parent

You may . . .

have postpartum depression and anxiety. It's not your fault and you aren't alone. Get help. Tell your provider how you feel. **Call or text 9-8-8** or call 1-833-TLC-MAMA (1-833-852-6262)

If you . . .

- Feel hopeless or like giving up
- Don't feel like you're in reality (you may see or hear things that others don't)
- Feel that you may hurt yourself, your baby, or your other kids

You need to **GET HELP NOW.**

- If baby is there, put them in their crib or another safe place or ask a friend or neighbor to hold them.
- **Call 9-1-1 for help right now.**
- **Or call 9-8-8 for support right now.**

If you need help right away, use the "find a breastfeeding counselor" link on the website to contact someone in your area.

La Leche League (LLL)

Learn about breastfeeding, pumping, and answers to common questions about nursing. Find a LLL leader near you or find your local LLL group. LLL meetings can be online or in person, are free of charge, and provide a safe place to ask questions or just be around other nursing families.

1-800-525-3243 or www.lllusa.org

WIC (Women, Infants, and Children program)

Learn about breastfeeding, pumping, and answers to common questions and problems. "Breastfeeding 101" has links to many helpful topics. You can also find links for partners, grandparents, and for how to sign up for the WIC program.

Wicbreastfeeding.fns.usda.gov

Milk sharing – Donor milk

Human Milk Banking Association of North America

Donate, find, or request breast milk for your baby.

www.hmbana.org

Peer-to-peer breastmilk sharing: There are many milk sharing groups on social media. Talk to your provider or breastfeeding counselor about the pros and cons of peer-to-peer milk sharing. Ask if they know of good resources for donor milk in your area.

Videos

Global Health Media

Click on "breastfeeding" to see all videos. Click on "All Audiences" and choose "Mothers and caregivers."

globalhealthmedia.org

International Breastfeeding Centre

ibconline.ca/breastfeeding-videos-english

Child abuse – *See violence*

Crying

The Fussy Baby Network

Someone to listen when baby won't stop fussing. Call to talk or leave a message and a trained support person will call you back.

1-888-431-2229 (English and Español)

National Center on Shaken Baby Syndrome

www.dontshake.org

App: The Period of PURPLE Crying – National Center on Shaken Baby Syndrome ▢

Learn about your baby's development and how it affects crying and sleep. Watch videos about why babies cry so much in the first months of life and when it might get better. Get tips for how to soothe baby and how to coping with your frustration.

Feeding baby

Breastfeeding – *See breastfeeding*

Formula feeding

American Academy of Pediatrics

www.healthychildren.org/English/ages
-stages/baby/formula-feeding/

Growth and development

Birth to 5! Watch me thrive!

helpmegrownational.org

Learn the signs. act early.

Learn all about your baby's development
from birth to age 5.

www.cdc.gov/ncbddd/actearly

App: Milestone Tracker

Learn about what to expect as your baby
grows in the first five years. Illustrations,
checklists, and videos show you what skills
to watch for. Use pictures and logs to track
baby's changes as they play, learn, speak,
act, and move. Includes resources for
parents.

cdc.gov/MilestoneTracker (English)

cdc.gov/Sigamos (Español)

App: The Wonder Weeks app

Use this app to learn about baby's big
developmental leaps (when they suddenly
learn new skills). Learn what happens
during a leap, when to expect them, and
how to help baby as they grow. Includes
videos, tracking logs, and parent forums.

thewonderweeks.com/the-wonder-weeks
-app

Zero to Three

Learn about baby's social, emotional, and
physical development from birth through
age 3. Get tips for how to support baby's

growth before and after they are born.
Find links for the Tribal Home Visiting
program.

www.zerotothree.org/for-families

Safety and injury prevention

Center for Disease Control and Prevention (CDC)

www.cdc.gov/parents/infants

Safe Kids

www.safekids.org

Check for recalls

All used baby items should be checked
for recalls. Here you can search for recalls
on car seats, cribs, swings, and other baby
gear all in one place. Click on "Search for
recalls" to find a search page for all kinds
of recalls.

www.recalls.gov

Car seats

Safe Kids

Learn about proper car seat use. Find a
free car-seat check near you or schedule
one online. Some local Safe Kids
coalitions offer free or low-cost seats, or
may know where to get one in your area.

www.safekids.org/car-seat

NHTSA

Learn about proper car seat use. Look up
the laws in your state. Register your car
seat for recalls or look up vehicle recalls.

www.nhtsa.gov/carseat

AAP

American Academy of Pediatrics offers lots of car seat and travel tips under "Safety and Prevention," click "on the go."

healthychildren.org

Safe sleep

CPSC

Learn about safe sleep, product testing, and how to make sure your used baby gear is safe to use. Register or look up recalls for baby items.

www.cpsc.gov/SafeSleep

Cribs for Kids

Learn all about safe sleep and making sure your baby's sleep space is safe. Tips and videos on lots of topics.

safesleepacademy.org/

If you need a safe crib for baby: cribsforkids.org/request-a-crib/

Safe to Sleep

Learn all about SIDS and other sleep-related deaths, and how to keep your baby safe.

Safetosleep.nichd.nih.gov

Vaccines for baby

CDC

www.cdc.gov/vaccines-children

Immunize.org

Vaccines for baby

www.vaccineinformation.org/infants-children

Support for parents

Healthy Families America

A family support worker visits you in your home (or another comfortable place) to offer support. It can be a time to just visit and play, or it can be a safe place to talk about hard things. They can help you find resources or get more help. Click on "families" or "find an HFA" to find a program near you.

www.healthyfamiliesamerica.org

Nurse-Family Partnership

A nurse visits you in your home to provide learning and support. Starts early in pregnancy (before 28 weeks) and goes until your baby is 2 years old. Call, text, or look on the website to find a NFP program near you. (English and Español)

1-844-637-6667 or

www.nursefamilypartnership.org

Parents as Teachers

A parent educator visits you in your home to provide learning and support, from pregnancy until kindergarten. Offers in-person and virtual support. Click on "find programs" to find one near you.

parentsasteachers.org

Substance use – Quitting tobacco, drugs, and alcohol

SAMHSA

Look for help for mental health or substance use. Learn about addiction and mental illness and how to find and pay for treatment.

1-800-662-4357 or findtreatment.gov

SMART Recovery Programs

Addiction recovery programs that use a our-step process to support those who have addictions. Also has groups for family and friends of people with addictions. Special programs for youth and teens, LGBTQIA+, military and first responders, and those dealing with addiction while in prison. Offers help by mobile app, blog, podcast, videos, and online resources.

smartrecovery.org

Smokefree

Learn about making a quit plan that works for you. Get support before, while, and after you quit. Offers help by phone, text, app, social media, and online.

smokefree.gov

Quitline

Support before, while, and after you quit smoking, vaping, or using tobacco. Quit coaches can listen, offer advice, and connect you with quit-smoking medicines and other resources.

1-800-QUIT-NOW (1-800-784-8669) English

1-855-DEJELO-YA (1-855-335-3569) Español

Violence and abuse

National Child Abuse Hotline

Learn the signs of abuse, how to report it, and get help. Find out what counts as abuse, how to protect your child, and what to expect if you make a report. Offers help to teens who are being hurt by their adults, too. Get support by phone, text, or online chat.

Call or text 1-800-422-4453 or chat at www.childhelphotline.org

National Domestic Violence Hotline

Learn about the signs of abuse and how to make a plan for safety. Find legal help and local resources. Offers help by phone, text, or chat.

1-800-799-7233 or text "START" to 88788

Chat online at www.thehotline.org

National Deaf Domestic Violence Hotline

Help for deaf, blind, or hard of hearing survivors

Video phone: 1-855-812-1001

Email: nationaldeafhotline@adwas.org

Instant messenger: DeafHotline

StrongHearts Native Helpline

Support for Native American and Alaska Native survivors

Call or text 1-844-762-8483 or chat online at strongheartshelpline.org

National Women's Law Center

Learn more about and get resources for problems with child care, school, harassment, health care, equality, poverty, and your job.

nwlc.org

Other Books to Check Out

These books may be longer and not as easy to read, but they are filled with great information that many people find helpful. Most should be available from your local library.

Pregnancy and birth

Pregnancy, Childbirth, and the Newborn – Penny Simkin PT, Janet Whalley BSN IBCLC, Ann Keppler MN, and others (2024)

Your Pregnancy and Childbirth Month to Month – American College of Obstetrics and Gynecology (2021)

Mayo Clinic's Guide to Healthy Pregnancy – Myra J. Wick MD PhD (2024)

The First-Time Parent's Childbirth Handbook – Stephanie Mitchell CNM MSN DNP (2021)

Nurture: A Modern Guide to Pregnancy, Birth, Early Motherhood – Erica Chidi (2017)

A Child is Born – Lennart Nilsson and Linda Forsell (2020)

The Simple Guide to Having a Baby – Janet Whalley RN BSN, Penny Simkin PT, and Ann Keppler RN MN (2016)

The Birth Partner – Penny Simkin PT and Melissa Cheyney PhD (2024)

When You're Expecting Twins, Triplets, or Quads – Dr. Barbara Luke and Tamara Eberlein (2017)

Baby care

Caring for Your Baby and Young Child, Birth to Age 5 – American Academy of Pediatrics (2024)

Baby 411: Your Baby, Birth to Age 1 – Ari Brown MD and Denise Fields (2022)

The Wonder Weeks: A Stress-Free Guide to Your Baby's Behavior – Hatty van de Rijt PhD, Frans Plooij PhD, and Xaviera Plas-Plooij (2019)

Breastfeeding

The Art of Breastfeeding – La Leche League International (2024)

Breastfeeding: Keep it Simple – Amy Spangler MN RN IBCLC (2019)

Glossary: Words to know

Abdomen – Your body between the chest and pelvis, where the stomach, uterus, and other organs are. Your belly.

Abortion – Ending of a pregnancy, which may be natural (miscarriage) or done by a doctor (induced).

Air Bag – A safety feature in vehicles that bursts out and provides cushion in a crash.

Amniocentesis – A test of the fluid inside the bag of waters, showing certain things about your unborn baby's health.

Amniotic fluid – Liquid in the amniotic sac.

Amniotic sac – The "bag of waters" inside the uterus, in which the baby grows.

Anesthesia – Various drugs used to reduce or eliminate pain.

Antibodies – Cells made in a person's body to fight disease.

Aspirin – A pain and fever reducer that should only be used in pregnancy if prescribed. Do not give to babies or use while breastfeeding.

Areola – The dark area around the nipple.

Bag of waters – The amniotic sac in which your baby grows inside the uterus.

Birth canal – Your vagina, the opening through which your baby will be born.

Birth control – Ways to keep from getting pregnant when you have sex. Examples: condom, diaphragm, pills, IUD.

Birth defect – Baby's health problem that happens before birth or during birth. May have lasting effects.

Blood pressure – The force of blood pumped by the heart through a person's blood vessels. High blood pressure means the heart is pumping extra hard.

Bloody show – A small amount of mucus and blood (the "mucus plug") that comes from your cervix before labor begins.

Braxton-Hicks contractions – Tightening and relaxing of the muscle of your uterus during the last few months of pregnancy.

Breech birth – Birth of a baby who is not head-down. (Often buttocks first.)

Calcium – A mineral in foods needed to make bones and teeth grow strong.

Calories – Energy in foods. Some kinds of foods have more calories than others.

Car seat – Safety seat proven to protect children from injury and death in a vehicle crash.

Certified Nurse-midwife – A nurse who delivers babies, who has been specially trained as a midwife and passed a national test.

Cervix – The neck (opening) of the uterus (womb). Your baby is pushed out through the cervix into the vagina during delivery.

Cesarean section – Surgical birth of a baby through a cut in the belly. Also called c-section.

Child safety seat – See car seat.

Circumcision – Surgery to take off the loose skin around the tip of a baby's penis.

Colostrum – The thin, yellowish milk made in late pregnancy and the first few days after birth.

Conception – The start of a baby forming. When a sperm meets an egg.

Condom – A rubber or latex tube with a closed end that is used during sex to prevent pregnancy and diseases that can be passed during sex. An external condom is put on the penis just before sex. An internal condom is put into the vagina or anus just before sex.

Constipation – When bowel movements are very hard and do not come regularly.

Contraception – See Birth control.

Contractions – The tightening of the muscle of your uterus.

Core – The main part of your body (chest, shoulders, abdomen, back).

C-section – See Cesarean section.

Development – The ways in which the baby's mind learns and the body grows and changes.

Diarrhea – Bowel movements that are very soft and watery and come more often than usual.

Digestion – The changing of your food in your mouth, stomach, and intestines for use by your body.

Dilation – The stretching open of the cervix during the first stage of labor.

Discharge – Liquid that comes out of your body, like blood or mucus from your vagina.

Doula – A person trained to help parents during and after delivery.

Drop – The sinking of the unborn baby down into the pelvis before birth begins.

Drugs – Many kinds of things that affect your body or feelings, such as medicines, or substances like alcohol, tobacco, or illegal (street) drugs.

Due date – The date when a baby is expected to be born.

Effacement – The thinning of the cervix during the first stage of labor.

Embryo – Word used for a tiny unborn baby during the first eight weeks of its growth.

Engagement – The sinking (dropping) of the uterus down into the pelvis before birth.

Engorgement – Hard and painful breasts when very full of milk.

Episiotomy – A cut made in the skin around the vagina to widen the opening and help the baby to be born.

Family physician or practitioner – A doctor who takes care of the health of people of all ages.

Family planning – Using birth control to choose when to avoid getting pregnant and when not to.

Fertility – The ability to conceive a child.

Fetal monitor – A machine that tells how the unborn baby's heart is beating, used to check the baby's health inside the uterus.

Fetus – Word used for the unborn baby, from 8 weeks to birth at about 40 weeks.

Fiber – A part of food that helps bowel movements be soft and regular.

Fontanelles – Soft spots in the skull of a newborn baby. They close slowly over many months.

Formula – Special milk for bottle-feeding. Made to be much like breast milk.

Genetic counseling – Help for people with health problems that may be passed down to their children.

Genetic defects – Health problems that are passed down from parent to child to grandchild through genetic matter in the cells.

Genitals – The penis or vulva.

Gestational diabetes – A type of diabetes that happens only in pregnancy. If untreated, it can be harmful for both parent and baby.

Group B streptococcus (GBS) – A type of bacteria ("strep") that can live in the vagina and can seriously harm a newborn baby.

Health care provider – A person trained to take care of people's health and illness (nurses, doctors, midwives).

Heartburn – A burning feeling in your chest caused by acid from your stomach going up into the esophagus (tube from mouth to stomach).

Hemorrhoids – Veins at your anus (opening where stool comes out) that get swollen and feel itchy or painful.

Hormones – Substances made by organs in the body that control how it works and feels.

Immune system – The body system that fights disease by making antibodies.

Immunization (vaccination, shot) – Delivery of a vaccine that helps the body make antibodies to fight against a disease.

Incubator – A covered bed used in the NICU. It keeps baby's temperature and oxygen just right.

Induce, induction – Start contractions with drugs or other means.

Infection – A sore or illness caused by germs that harm your body.

Intact penis – A penis that hasn't been circumcised.

Iron – A mineral in foods that helps your blood carry oxygen to your baby's body.

Isolette – See Incubator.

Kangaroo care – Holding baby with their bare skin on your bare skin. Also called skin-to-skin care.

Kegel – An exercise to strengthen the pelvic muscles below your bladder.

Labor – The work your uterus does to open the cervix and push the baby down into the birth canal.

LATCH system – Lower Anchors and Tethers for Children; a way of installing a car seat in a vehicle using special connectors on the car seat and anchors in the vehicle.

Lactation specialist – A person with special training and knowledge about breastfeeding (lactation).

Lanugo – Soft, short hair growing on the body of a fetus and newborn baby.

Medication – Drugs (medicines) that a doctor prescribes for you or that you can buy at a drug store.

Menstrual period – The bloody lining of the uterus that comes out of the vagina each month. A period.

Midwife – A person who helps women have their babies. (Not a doctor.)

Miscarriage (spontaneous abortion) – When an embryo or fetus is born too young to survive (before 20 weeks).

Mood disorder – An emotional illness or condition that can affect everyday life.

Morning sickness – The feeling of nausea (needing to vomit) or vomiting that happens early in pregnancy.

Mucus plug – The thick blob of mucus that fills the cervix during pregnancy.

Multiple pregnancy – Twins, triplets, or more babies born at the same time.

Neonatal Intensive Care Unit (NICU) – The hospital nursery for preemies or those with serious medical problems.

Nurse-midwife – A nurse with special training to deliver babies.

Nurse practitioner – A nurse with special training to do some aspects of health care, working with a doctor.

Nursing – Another word for breastfeeding.

Nutrients – Things in foods that keep you healthy.

Obstetrician-Gynecologist – A doctor who provides reproductive health care before, during, and after pregnancy and birth. An obstetrician specializes in prenatal care and child birth. A gynecologist specializes in care of the uterus, vagina, and other female organs.

Pediatrician – A doctor who takes care of children's health.

Pelvic exam – A way for your doctor or nurse midwife to check your vagina and uterus by pressing on your belly and reaching up inside your vagina, and by looking inside.

Pelvis – Your hip bones inside which your uterus sits. Your vagina (birth canal) goes through a wide opening in these bones.

Perinatal – The time before and after a baby's birth.

Perineum – The skin and muscles around the opening of the vagina. Also called the pelvic floor.

Period – A short word for menstrual period.

Postpartum – The period of time after pregnancy or birth.

Placenta – An organ that forms in the uterus after conception, attached to baby's umbilical cord. The placenta connects to the uterus. It carries oxygen and nutrients to baby and takes waste away.

Preemie – A short term for a preterm infant.

Pregnancy – The 40 weeks when a baby is growing inside the uterus.

Pregnancy-induced hypertension (PIH) – High blood pressure during pregnancy. May lead to preeclampsia if not treated.

Prenatal – During pregnancy.

Prescription – An order for medicine from your doctor.

Preterm (premature) – A baby born early, before the 37th week of pregnancy.

Protein – Substances in food that make your body grow well and work properly.

Reflexes – Movements of the body that happen automatically.

Reflux – Acid from the stomach that backs up into the esophagus (tube from the mouth to the stomach).

Sexually transmitted infection (STI) – A disease passed by sharing fluids from the mouth, vagina, penis, or anus. A sexually transmitted disease (STD). Common STIs are chlamydia, gonorrhea, herpes, and syphilis.

Spinal cord – The main nerve in the body that goes up the middle of the spine or backbone. It connects the brain to the rest of the body.

Stillbirth – When a baby dies before or during birth (after 20 weeks).

Stool – A bowel movement. Poop.

Sudden infant death syndrome (SIDS) – Death of a sleeping baby when all other causes have been ruled out.

Swaddling – Wrapping a newborn baby snugly in a thin blanket for comfort.

Symptoms – Changes in your body or how you feel (like pain, itching, or bleeding). These help your provider know what health problem you have.

Temporal artery thermometer: A thermometer that senses temperature from the artery under the forehead skin.

Trimester – A three-month time period. A full pregnancy has three trimesters.

Tympanic thermometer: A thermometer that senses temperature from the ear opening.

Ultrasound – Special tool used to see inside your body to find out how your unborn baby is doing or growing.

Umbilical cord – The long tube that attaches the placenta to the unborn baby's body at the navel (belly button). It carries oxygen and nutrients in to baby and carries waste away.

Uterus – The womb, the organ in which an unborn baby grows.

Vaccine – Substance given to immunize against disease. (See Immunizations.)

Vagina – The opening to the birth canal. Menstrual blood or discharge come out here. A penis (or fingers, etc.) can go inside here for sex. Can stretch open for baby to come out in a vaginal birth.

Vaginal birth – A baby is born by moving down through the cervix and birth canal and out the vagina.

Varicose veins – Blue, swollen veins that itch or ache, that often occur in the legs during pregnancy.

VBAC – Vaginal Birth After a Cesarean.

Vernix – Grayish-white, cheese-like cream covering the skin of a newborn baby.

Vomiting – Throwing up stomach contents.

Vulva – The mound and outer labia (lips) that cover the vagina. The part of the genitals you can see when the labia are closed.

Well-baby, Well-child checkup – Regular health visits for babies and children who are not ill. Checkups cover health, development, immunizations, and screening tests.

WIC (Women, Infants, and Children) Program – A healthy nutrition program for low-income people in pregnancy and postpartum, and children up to age 5.

Index